To my beloved grandmothers, Phil He Lee (이필혜) and Ha Soon Kim (김하순), for planting seeds of wisdom and nourishing me to become a giving tree.

To my parents, Yoo Jong Yoon and June Yoon, who have shown me that anything is possible with deep devotion and unconditional love.

To my sisters, Sara Yoon and Joanne Yoon, thank you for being a source of love and light in my life.

To my teachers and mentors, your collective kindness and influence have inspired me to expand my heart to others and pay it forward for the rest of my life.

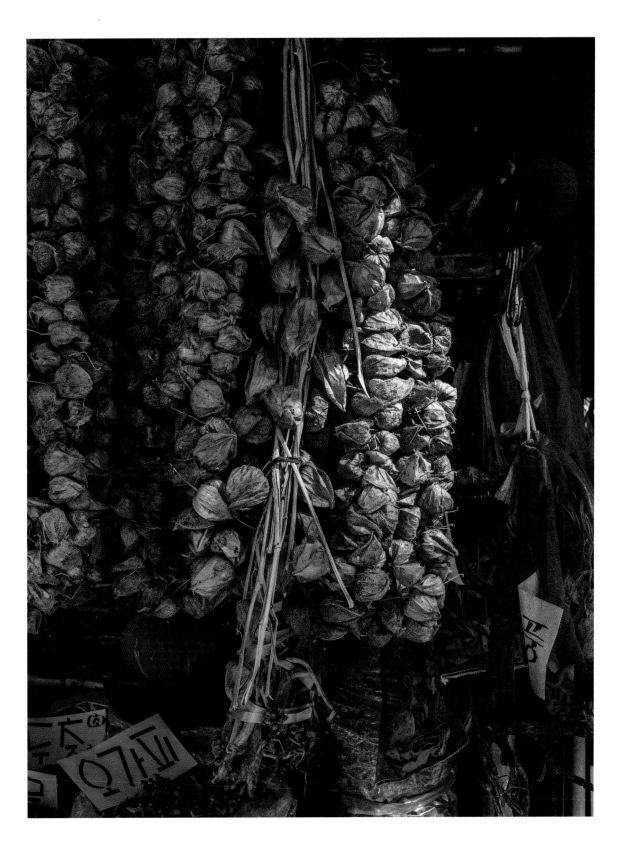

CONTENTS

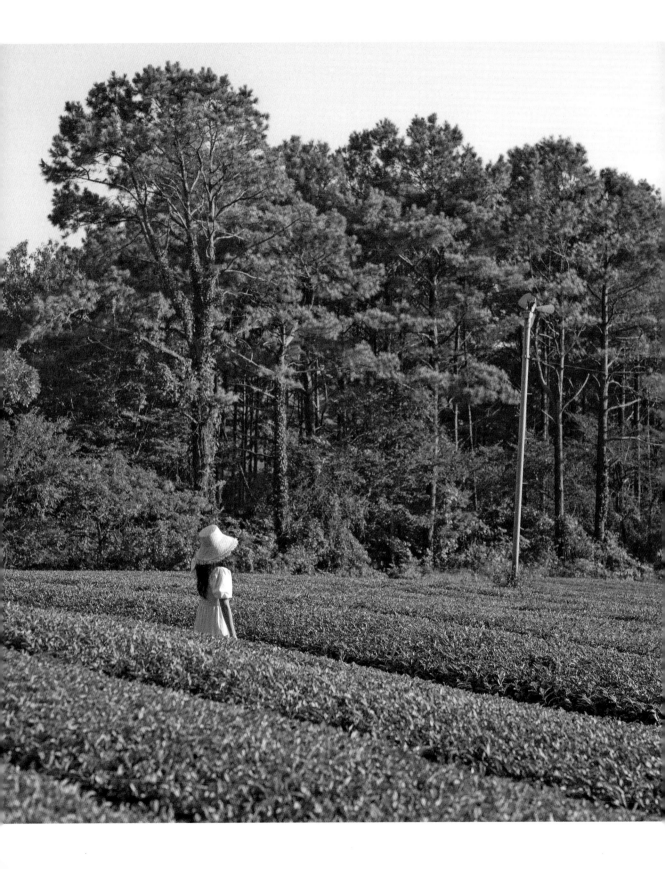

INTRODUCTION

Grace is my English name. 사은 is my Korean name, and the characters represent love and grace. As a Korean American, I had the privilege of being taught to embrace both cultures, and my journey into herbalism begins with my ancestral roots.

My paternal grandmother (할머니) was a farmer in Paju, South Korea. She was a productive woman, raising six children on her own. She also was a midwife to the local village and managed a commercial farm while actively being involved in her local community. A true matriarch, her rustic, leathery hands always reminded me of the labor of love that is harvesting beautiful herbs and vegetables. She never cared about her external appearance. No manicures or perms for this woman—she lived organically. She was Mother Nature.

My maternal grandmother (외할머니), by contrast, loved the elegant things of life. Married to a major after the Korean War, she wore custom-made dresses and pearl necklaces, played tennis, and lived on a vineyard in the middle of Seoul. She was happy and satisfied (행복해). Then, her world changed when my grandfather had a sudden heart attack. She became a widow with six children to support and no vocational skills. Soon after, a truck hit my grandmother while she was driving and she became partially paralyzed on the left side of her body. It was through the power of acupuncture and herbal medicine that she was able to regain strength and movement. From her own healing experience, she devoted her life to Eastern medicine and studied to become a healer.

When my parents emigrated to the US, my dad was a college student and my mom, who graduated from art school in Korea, worked at a local floral shop. Soon after, my grandmothers joined my parents to live the American dream. My sisters and I now were surrounded by immense love, especially from our grandmothers.

Both of my grandmothers taught me their knowledge in Eastern medicine and Korean secrets to holistic healing through plants. America was a foreign place for them, so they spent their time at local parks foraging the land. The park near their home oddly resembled the fields in Korea. They would come back with bags of mugwort, acorns, pecans, and dandelion root, and they would make delicious Korean cuisine or herbal soaps.

My paternal grandmother longed for her farm back in Korea, and while she was walking to the park, she came across a local landfill covered with trash. For some, it was just garbage, but she saw its hidden potential. Each day, she would pick up trash, and after several months, what *was* a landfill became her garden. There, she invited a group of Korean grandmothers and created a community garden for people to grow vegetables. She was a woman of few words, and her love was shown by her actions.

MY PATH TO HERBALISM

I had chronic health issues as a child. At the age of six, I had symptoms such as high fevers and difficulty breathing, and I was misdiagnosed many times. It was a stressful time for me and my family to navigate the American medical system. We turned to my grandmother, who was an Eastern medicine doctor, for help. Acupuncture and herbal remedies enabled my body to heal naturally. My shortness of breath and fevers disappeared, and I had energy and vitality. I had my internal life force back, my Qi. Through this experience, I realized the importance of health, nutrition, and growing my own plant medicine at an early age. I felt fortunate to have grandmothers who practiced Eastern medicine and herbalism.

And my chronic pain became my saving grace. Fast-forward to 2018. I was walking through an herbal market in South Korea, and I was reminded of my childhood illness. I asked myself, "Why aren't these herbal remedies as accessible in America?" We are one of the most prosperous countries in the world, yet we are going through a healthcare and food crisis, and we are not taking preventive measures commonly practiced in Korea.

Since birth, our bodies were created to fight disease naturally through nutrition and a healthy, balanced lifestyle. Our ancestors foraged plants out of necessity and made natural medicine to prevent and cure disease. Now, we live in a sedentary and artificial world that is ruining our health and longevity by consuming processed foods and prescription medications and destroying our ecosystem.

But what if there was a natural solution that our ancestors passed on to us that would help us relieve our pain? My understanding of the problems in America led me to share these effective Korean remedies and preventive practices with the West. Throughout this book, you will learn about herbs that offer certain vitamins and minerals to help balance your Qi. I share herbal recipes and remedies that are relevant to the seasons and our constitution. This book offers ancient Korean herbal wisdom with the modern world—starting with our Qi.

We are all from a garden.

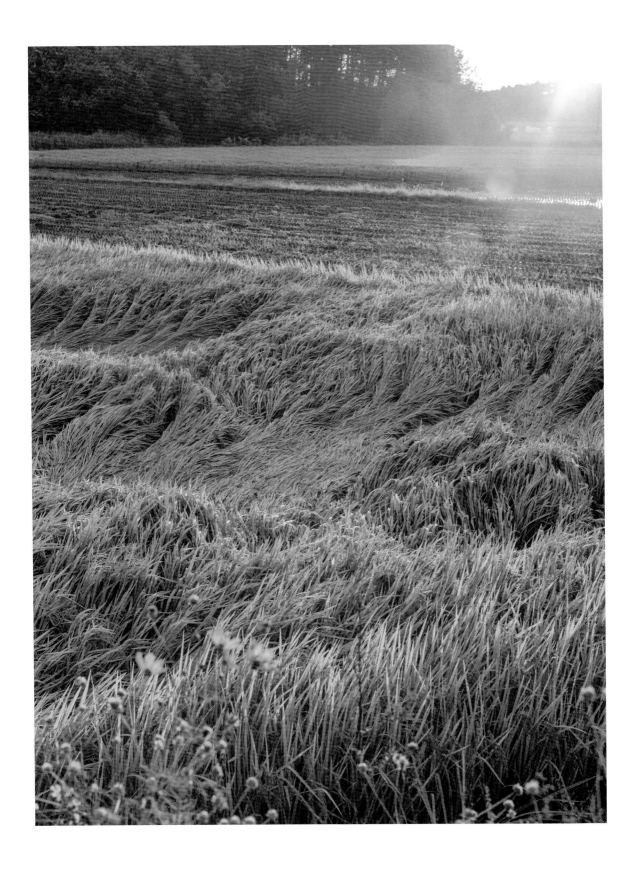

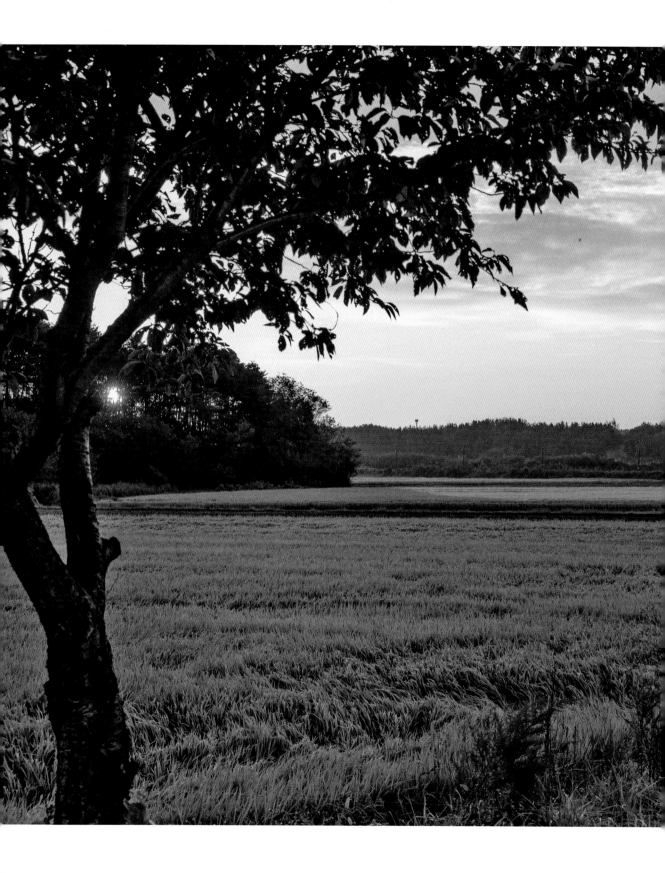

1

THE QI OF LIFE

기의 삶 [gisalm]

Born as a caterpillar, it's our time to grow—
Protected underground.
Our silky cocoon.

Internal changes
The world has yet to see

Metamorphosis . . .
weeks,
months,
years.

Compound eyes, wings to fly.
Fly high
Butterfly.

As herbalists, we are like butterflies. We are grounded humans, yet our curiosity transforms our hands so they can produce beautiful herbal mixtures. The remedies we create are healing yet sometimes time-consuming and laborious. When we make herbal foods, body care, or plant medicine, when we pull roots out of the soil or pick fruit from a tree, we are connecting our Qi, the vital life force in us, with Mother Nature.

Everything under the sun and moon is composed of Qi, and time has a way of showing the alchemy of life through Qi. Halmuni (할머니), my paternal grandmother, would take a walk into the woods and discover time in the Eastern way. A gargantuan oak tree with a wide trunk and many branches sprouting leaves and acorns stood in front of us. As she foraged acorns from the ground, she placed one in my palm and said that we, like every tree, start life as a small seed.

Each acorn contains one seed that may or may not grow into an oak tree. Seeds come in all shapes and sizes, and they are dispersed in different ways: Some cross-pollinate by insects, others are carried by the wind. But, most important, all seeds need proper nutrients to survive and grow into a giving tree.

TREE OF QI

Before spring rain,
A baby seed.

After spring rain,
A baby sprout.

Two become three
As a family tree.

We are here.

Once your roots take hold, an emergence begins.
Breaking through soil, strong roots planted
To uphold the world.

The seed is planted at our birth. In this vulnerable stage, the first root bursts through the seed and anchors itself into the soil to absorb water. Then, germination begins, and a shoot becomes a seedling. This time is critical, for the seedling will either emerge or rot just below the surface, and the stem will be most vulnerable to disease and hungry animals.

Once a seedling becomes a sapling, it may grow quickly but hasn't fully reached maturity. The young trunk is flexible, and the bark is smooth, but it cannot grow fruit and flowers yet. At this stage, the sapling is immature and unable to produce seeds. When a tree is fully mature, it is able to produce its own fruit, flowers, or nuts and reproduce and disperse its seeds. Now, it is a vital member of the ecosystem. An oak tree can live and produce acorns for twenty to two hundred years, longer than most other trees. As the tree slowly decays and dies, it gives to the biodiversity of the world around it by providing a home to insects and fungi as well as shelter to small creatures.

We all play a role in contributing to our communities and environment. Another contribution a tree gives to the beauty of the world is providing the wood for musical instruments such as a violin. Made from strong willow, the violin accompanied me through the stanzas of my life as soulful therapy. Music was my shelter, and as I play my violin, I'm reminded of the tree that gifted me with the medium to share melodies with others.

Grandma saw the life of a tree as Qi—a cyclical thread that connects all beings and governs all things in heaven and earth. Qi is the common denominator of all things from an acorn seed to the total energy of the universe. The Qi of the sun, rain, and every person living on this Earth are necessary elements to produce healthy soil, which anchors the roots of a sustaining tree.

We cannot see or define Qi, but we can feel and experience Qi when we expand our hearts and minds.

HERBAL ALCHEMIST: THE EASTERN WAY

Using herbs is energetic, and to be our own herbal alchemist, it is essential to understand our Eastern ancestry. In Asia, our ancestors passed on three spiritual philosophies or religions that Koreans mainly practice—Taoism, Buddhism, and Confucianism. Although Eastern medicine is rooted in Taoist philosophy, Koreans have evolved their own methodology of Eastern medicine that also combines Confucius and Buddhist theories into their herbal practice. Each philosophy takes a spiritual approach to life, so it is essential to have fresh eyes as we open our hearts and minds to a new way of thinking.

MOON EYES

Grandma said to keep my eyes in the shape of crescent moons.
Keep smiling even when times are hard.
The moon's reflection on water is the reflection of your heart.

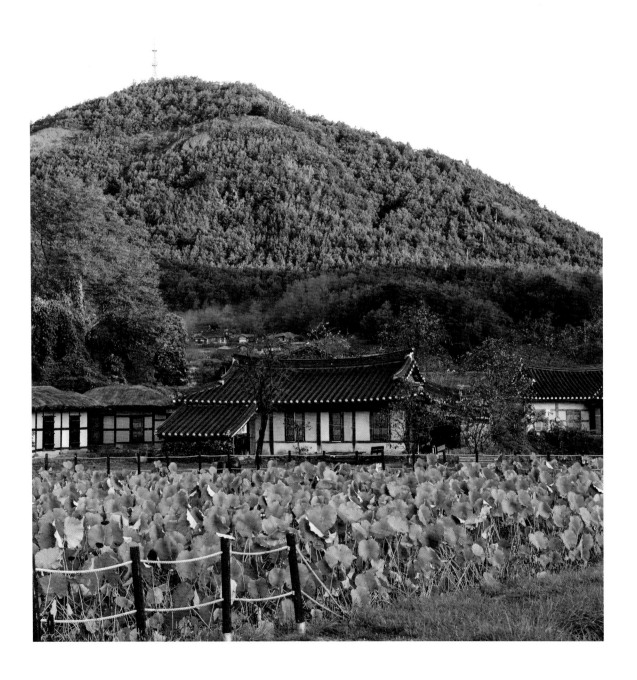

BALANCE IS QI: YIN AND YANG

While Qi is vital energy, we must consider the energetic qualities of yin and yang that are used to describe relationships, movements, patterns, and change. Life is a constant balance of yin and yang, a complementary dependence that is necessary for two polar states to live in harmony. Similar to riding an ocean wave, we cannot control the wave but allow it to naturally flow. Growing rice is yang, and reaping rice is yin. Whenever there is darkness, soon light will appear.

Experience Yin and Yang

Experiencing nature on a daily basis will enhance your senses to the energetic qualities of yin and yang. Begin by detaching yourself from any type of technology. We want to simplify our lives and flow freely. Wear loose-fitting clothes and comfortable shoes or no shoes. Bring a notebook and a writing utensil to write or draw your thoughts and feelings. Make sure you apply sunscreen as we always want to protect our skin from the sun.

I usually wear a flowy dress with sandals and carry a crossbody pouch that contains colored pencils, a pen, a small notepad, a pocket loupe (a magnifying lens), and tweezers. Once I find a spot to sit, I take off my shoes and let the grass or dirt tickle my toes. If the sun rays are strong, I usually find shade under a tree to protect my sensitive skin.

Take a stroll to the nearest garden or woods and be with nature. When we are outdoors, we feel and hear the wind's secrets. Listen to the direction of the birds while closing your eyes. Be in this moment for a few minutes. Then, look out and truly see the miracles of the plants growing from the soil or the leaves providing shade.

Occasionally, I will take out my loupe and observe the intricate details of a budding flower or a leaf of an herb or tree. Does the flower have a stigma, style, and ovary? Does it have a filament and anther? Does it have both a carpel and stamen? By using a loupe, we can see if a leaf's venation is palmate, parallel, pinnate, reticulate, or arcuate. When we see and understand the intricacies of a

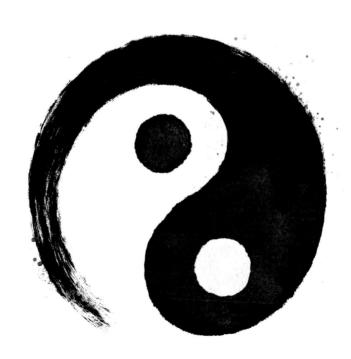

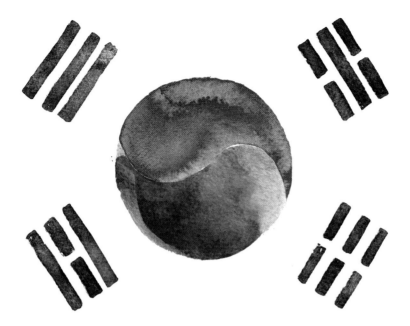

plant's anatomy and evolution and how it is similar to the evolution of people, our connection to nature deepens. It is the path of discovery.

Breathe in the air and expand your lungs. Cherish this moment and whatever you are going through and feeling. Give yourself permission to take the time to respect what you see, hear, feel, breathe, and taste.

Art is one of the best ways to connect with our environment. I often touch the trunk of a tree or stroke a leaf as I sing songs to heal my soul. On other days, I write poetry or sketch a plant depending on what I'm feeling, seeing, or hearing. An organoleptic practice of trying herbs is also a great way to deepen our taste buds.

Before picking a plant, give thanks to Mother Earth for providing us with the plant. Giving gratitude for the precious plant that Mother Nature has created for us will help us to be mindful whenever we harvest. Conscious harvesting will influence our hands to pick what we *need* and not harvest in excess. Sometimes, we take things for granted because we are blind to appreciate the basic necessities that Mother Earth has given us such as the air we breathe, the water to quench our thirst, and the plants that give us nutrients and wisdom.

Respect is an important quality in Korean culture as we honor our elders and ancestors with deep respect for what they have sacrificed for us. The biodiversity of plants that surround us has been passed on by nature and by the hands of native and indigenous people, so it is important to honor our ancestors for what they have done.

Once we harvest the amount we need and taste the herb, we can ask ourselves if the plant is astringent, bitter, or mucilaginous. What parts of the plants can we use to make medicine? What are the energetic ways of this plant? It is important to practice using our five senses to gather and bridge the world around us. It deepens our joy and closely connects our consciousness to Mother Earth.

We are all part of a family, and herbs are no different. Each herb is a member of a plant family, and drawing the herb in our journal is one of the best ways to identify and learn the herb we harvested. When we draw the fine details of the roots, leaves, stems, and sometimes flowers, we can identify family patterns and narrow down which family the plant is from. Thistles are all disk florets. Dandelions are all ray florets. Every plant has a unique botanical name, and there are thousands of plant species worldwide, so it may seem daunting at first to try to identify the plant, but first enjoy the process of getting to feel the plant and draw the beautiful details of it.

YIN-YANG ANCESTRAL TWINE

Yin, mysterious darkness of feminine energy like the moon's soft reflection on a river
Yang, illuminating light of masculine energy like the sun's clarity in exposing the mountains

Today, a brand-new moon
Tomorrow, a brand-new sun

The lightness of a dandelion is yin
The heaviness of a stone is yang
Take my hand and feel the Earthly soil of yin
Lift my arms and reach the Heavenly clouds of yang

Inside and down when traditions and ancestry fades
Outside and up as culture and tribes revive
Ancestral twine

Accepting and surrendering what is to come, yin
Willing to take a chance to fulfill our heart's desire, yang

Peace is yin
Hope is yang

Finding your place and your reason in this life can often be divided into night and day. There will be inactive yin seasons, like the fall and winter, and active yang seasons, like spring and summer. Taking the time to sit patiently and let the universe reveal the mysteries of life will bring us peace and wisdom.

YIN-YANG ENERGY IN TRIGRAMS

Similar to the depths of the earth and the peaks of the mountains, any yin or yang aspect can be further hewed into yin and yang. Trigrams are symbols of the cycles of yin and yang energy in all things. The eight trigrams—Heaven, Earth, Lake, Mountain, Fire, Water, Thunder, and Wind—represent the forces of nature.

Yang energy is a continuous line, and yin energy is a split line. Yin and yang mutually create each other.

Lao Tzu, the founder of Taoism, described the harmonious and transformational changes of yin and yang in *Tao Teh Ching*:

> *Being and nonbeing produce each other;*
> *Difficult and easy complete each other;*
> *Long and short construct each other;*
> *High and low distinguish each other;*
> *Sound and voice harmonize each other;*
> *Front and back follow each other.*
>
> *In order to contract,*
> *It is necessary first to expand.*
> *In order to weaken,*
> *It is necessary first to strengthen.*
> *In order to destroy,*
> *It is necessary first to promote.*
> *In order to grasp,*
> *It is necessary first to give.*

Although yin and yang are different, they depend on each other and cannot be separated. For example, temperature cannot be measured from the yin and yang of cold and hot.

YIN AND YANG AND THE EIGHT TRIGRAMS

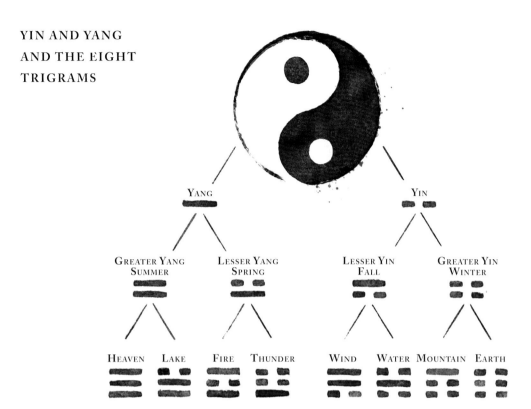

It's akin to the relationship between nature and people, where trees give us oxygen and nutrients from their branches and leaves. We are in living partnership with the earth, similar to the way most plants form symbiotic relationships. The fungi help roots of plants extend and reach to obtain water and nutrients that might not be available to the plant.

Humans have a responsibility to be conscious of our ecological footprint and care for Mother Earth. Nature is an organic process, and as changes occur, yin and yang are always supporting, repairing, and transforming into each other.

SEOUL NATION

As we take a deeper look into Korean ancestry, the elements of the South Korean flag, called Taegukgi (태극기), symbolize the dual yin and yang, or positive and negative, forces of nature, humanity, and society.

The white field of the flag, a traditional color in Korean culture, represents the peace and purity that our land provides. On the Eastern side of the Asian continent, located between China and Japan, Korea (called Hanguk, 한국) is surrounded by three seas: the Yellow Sea, East China Sea, and Sea of Japan. Our land is a small yet prominent peninsula, largely mountainous with valleys and coastal plains, and is often called the Land of High Mountains and Sparkling Streams.

Korea was once the Land of Tigers, home to a large population of majestic tigers, even the rare white tiger that is a sacred spirit animal of wisdom. Tigers appear frequently in Korean folklore, and as you continue reading this book, you will learn a few and understand the spirit of the tiger.

Shaded in blue and red, yin (also called eum, 음) and yang are located in the center, symbolizing our people, the Korean race. Koreans are passionate, peaceful, and loyal people. We have suffered through many wars in the past and have been colonized and repressed, but our people have never started wars with other countries. Our resilient nature has made us productive, and ambition has given us dreams for a better future. The hardships of war change people and generations. Grandma never spoke about the Korean War, but I could tell by looking into her eyes and working hands that she faced hardship, sadness, and tragedy. Through her deep pain and love, she endured and paved the way for the next generation to thrive and give back to our community.

Family is the nucleus of our society as Korean culture practices Confucian ideology—giving deep respect and honor to our ancestors and elders is ingrained in our culture. Each fall during the harvest moon, an ancient national holiday takes place where families gather to honor our ancestors. Special dishes, such as foraged chestnuts or freshly picked persimmons, are prepared and presented in front of a shrine for our ancestors. Bowing to our elders and ancestors is a ritual that brings honor and respect to the past generation. In the mountains, you will see burial mounds as Koreans buried their ancestors vertically under these mounds. We walk around our ancestors' burial mounds, bow twice, and offer spirit food and drink. The practice of remembering our ancestors is a beautiful ritual that commemorates the love and pain that our ancestors experienced to further each generation.

BALANCE IN THE UNIVERSE

As yin is to yang, there are negative and positive energetic qualities to humanity. The perpetual changing forces of good and evil, active and passive, masculine and feminine, and light and darkness are always constant. Asking ourselves each day if we are more yin or yang or both is a good way to energetically check in with ourselves. How are you feeling right now? Really dive in to your five senses to feel. Express your thoughts or feelings through art, writing, music, meditation, or movement.

The four trigrams on each corner represent our nation. Further hewed, the trigrams represent natural elements (air, wood, water, fire), celestial body (heaven, sun, moon, earth), four seasons (spring, summer, autumn, winter), four virtues (humanity, justice, respect, intelligence), family members (father, mother, daughter, son), and cardinal directions (north, south, east, west). The trigrams show the constant cycles of yin and yang energy in nature, the celestial body, the seasons, virtues, our family, and cardinal directions. Throughout the book, we will learn the deeper meanings of each trigram, which all circle back to Qi.

TRIGRAMS OF THE KOREAN FLAG

	☰ 건 GEON	☷ 곤 GON	☲ 리 LEE	☵ 감 GAM
Natural element	Air	Wood	Fire	Water
Celestial body	Heaven	Earth	Sun	Moon
Seasons	Spring	Summer	Autumn	Winter
Family member	Father	Mother	Daughter	Son
Cardinal direction	East	West	South	North

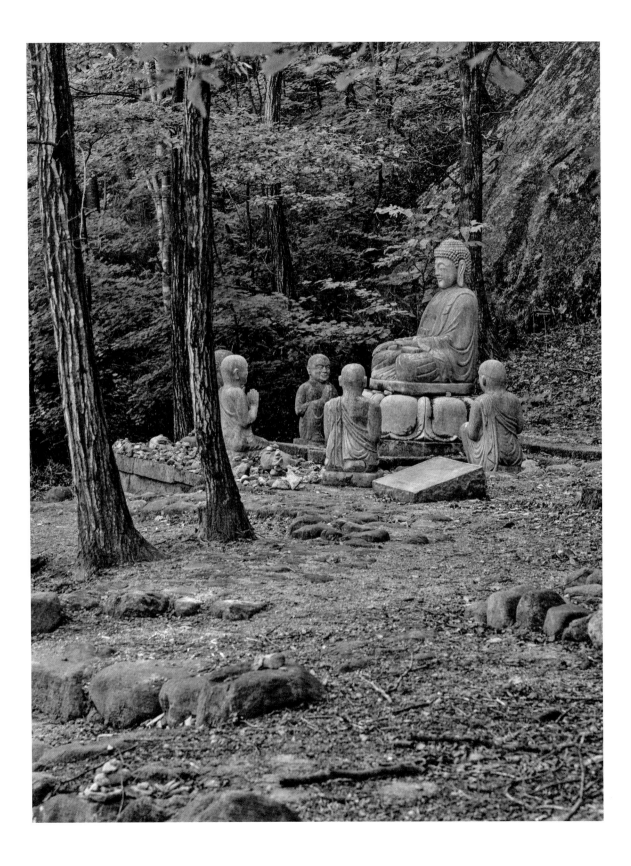

THE POWER OF FIVE

Herbs and medicine have the same root—providing nutrients, restoring our health, and balancing our Qi. A traditional Korean meal includes various herbal dishes formed by energetic qualities of yin and yang that create the five elements in Korean cuisine (wood, fire, earth, metal, and water).

The five elemental foods are selected mindfully. They include a spectrum of five cardinal colors (obangsaek, 오방색):

- Blue represents trees in the woods.
- Red represents fire.
- Yellow represents the earth.
- White represents metal.
- Black represents the sea.

The balance of yin and yang is similar to cold kimchi complemented by hot seaweed soup. Foods from the mountains are harmonious with foods from the sea. The sea provides us with water and shapes everything in the universe, including our health and longevity.

All these elemental colors are necessary for a healthy and prosperous life. When experiencing a Korean meal, notice the five cardinal colors. For example, yellow sautéed ginkgo nuts, white bellflower root mixed with Korean red pepper flakes, steamed spinach sprinkled with sesame seeds, pickled radish and carrot, fermented kimchi full of nutrients and flavor, and multigrain rice. Some of the most popular Korean dishes, such as bibimbap rice bowl, kimbap rolls, and japchae, represent obangsaek cuisine.

Notice the different colors you are eating. Does your meal have five cardinal colors? Are you eating wood, fire, earth, metal, and sea? If not, allow yourself to ask why you are not eating the colors of nature. Our food is our daily medicine.

Each element also corresponds to one of five flavors (sour, bitter, sweet, spicy, and salty) and to an emotion (anger, joy, worry, sadness, and fear), and the emotions further branch out to corresponding organs in our body. The wood element is sour. The fire element is bitter. The earth element is sweet. The metal element is spicy. The water element is salty.

The sweetness of the earth may bring a calming and hydrating effect when we are in a state of worry. The strong spicy flavors may activate our Qi and alleviate our sadness. The bitter flavors may inflame a joy in our heart and stimulate the central nervous system. Trying the five elemental flavors during different seasons will help balance your yin-yang organs as our body is constantly changing.

If one of our organs is ill or imbalanced, the food of the same element can help to repair the damage to that organ. Here are a few examples of elemental herbs that we can use to bring back balance in our organs.

WOOD HERBS FOR LIVER AND GALLBLADDER	FIRE HERBS FOR HEART AND SMALL INTESTINE	EARTH HERBS FOR STOMACH AND PANCREAS	METAL HERBS FOR LUNGS AND LARGE INTESTINE	WATER HERBS FOR BLADDER AND KIDNEYS
Jujubes	Lotus seeds	Astragalus	Scallion	Ginseng
Goji berries	Cayenne	Ginger	Garlic	Holy basil
Chrysanthemum flowers	Beets	Persimmon	Tangerine peel	Rehmannia root
Peony root	Cherries	Cinnamon	White onion	Black sesame seed
Artichoke	Lychee berries	Pumpkin	Pear	Pomegranate
Spinach		Curcumin		

FIVE ELEMENTS
Yak Sik Dong Won

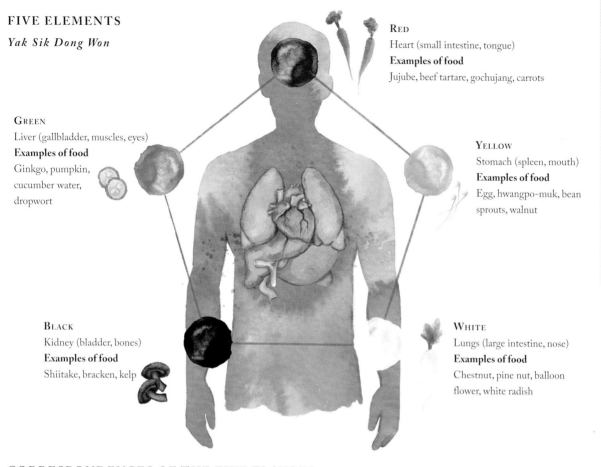

RED
Heart (small intestine, tongue)
Examples of food
Jujube, beef tartare, gochujang, carrots

GREEN
Liver (gallbladder, muscles, eyes)
Examples of food
Ginkgo, pumpkin, cucumber water, dropwort

YELLOW
Stomach (spleen, mouth)
Examples of food
Egg, hwangpo-muk, bean sprouts, walnut

BLACK
Kidney (bladder, bones)
Examples of food
Shiitake, bracken, kelp

WHITE
Lungs (large intestine, nose)
Examples of food
Chestnut, pine nut, balloon flower, white radish

CORRESPONDENCES OF THE FIVE FLAVORS

ELEMENT	FLAVOR	EMOTION	YIN-YANG ORGANS
Wood	Sour	Anger	Yin: Liver / Yang: Gallbladder
Fire	Bitter	Joy	Yin: Heart / Yang: Small intestine
Earth	Sweet	Worry	Yin: Spleen / Yang: Stomach
Metal	Spicy	Sadness	Yin: Lungs / Yang: Large intestine
Water	Salty	Fear	Yin: Kidneys / Yang: Bladder

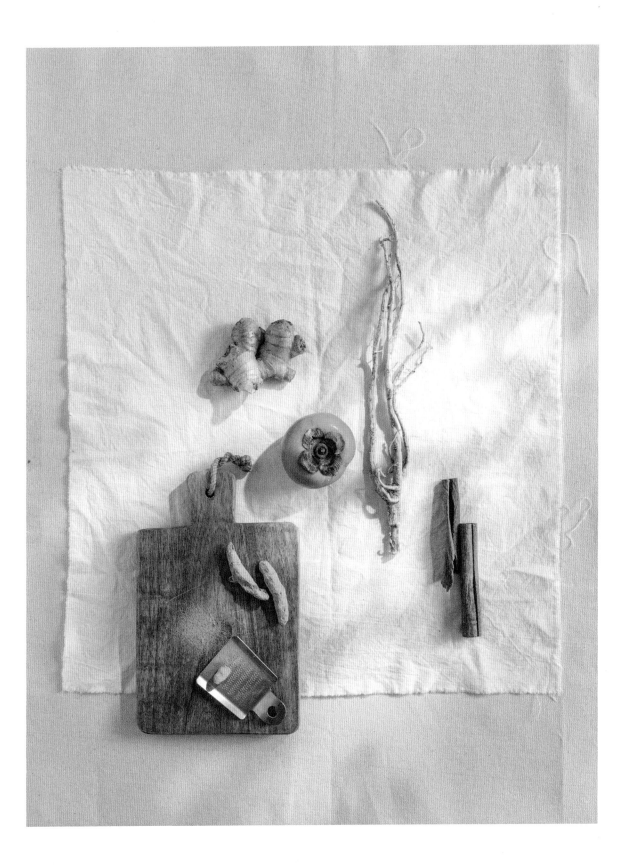

Traditionally, an herbal dish is prepared based on how the flavors and colors contradict and adapt with one another. For a balanced yin-yang dish, it is necessary to understand this harmony. Yin-producing foods and herbs are moistening, nourishing, or alkaline-dense. Yang herbs, on the other hand, are active in nature, and they increase metabolism and acidity. For example, a black sesame porridge is a yin food, and it is served with kimchi, which is yang, to ensure balance.

If yang is high in your body, food that is yin should be taken to bring harmony. If a person is high in yin, an incremental increase in the yang food will create balance. This requires time and intuition to understand your body and what it needs and a steady progression to feel if it is good for your body.

The balance between flavors, our emotions, our organs, and our environment is a perennial way of life. Balancing yin and yang is an important part of optimizing the quality of our lives as well as expanding our time to live at our highest potential.

The five elements of metal, fire, earth, wood, and water correspond to the five flavors of sour, bitter, sweet, spicy, and salty, which ties to our five emotions of anger, joy, worry, sadness, and fear, connecting our organ systems from the liver, heart, stomach, lungs, to kidneys. Without elements, flavors, emotions, and our organs, there would be no life. There would be no Qi.

The elements used in broth that have sweet, spicy, neutral, and cool profiles support their effect in detoxing the body and also have been shown to help relieve hangovers. Hangover relief is related to the breakdown of acetaldehyde from alcohol and intake of fluids and electrolytes. Our Korean ancestors were able to develop such versatile and effective food from using Eastern philosophy and the native herbs that were passed down through generations.

ELEMENTS TO CREATE NOURISHING BROTHS WITH YIN-YANG FLAVORS

ELEMENTS	YIN-YANG FLAVORS
Bean sprouts	Sweet and neutral
Radish	Sweet, spicy, and cool
Cabbage	Sweet and cool
Scallion	Spicy and warm
Sea trout/kelt	Salty and cold
Chive	Spicy and warm
Taro stem	Spicy and neutral
Curled mallow	Sweet and cold
Watercress	Sweet, spicy, and cool
Ox	Sweet and warm
Anchovy	Sweet and neutral
Corbicula clam	Sweet, salty, and cold
Pollack	Sweet and neutral
Blowfish	Sweet and warm

SPECTRUM OF FIVE RICE ROLL

김밥 [kimbap]

Halmuni prepared kimbap by rolling rice with fermented or steamed herbs and vegetables in dried laver seaweed and packed it in my lunchbox. My classmates would surround me during lunch wondering what Grandma made for me this time. The curious kids would try to trade their PB&J sandwich for a couple kimbap rolls, but it didn't make sense to exchange my colorful nutrient-dense rolls for a piece of bread with jam and peanuts.

Kimbap, one of Korea's most popular dishes, represents the five elements. The beauty of making kimbap is the different variations of rice, herbs, vegetables, and meats based on our dietary preferences.

As good things take time, preparing all the herbal fillings requires some patience. The multigrain rice gives it a delicious and rich taste along with the herbs and vegetables containing vitamins and antioxidants. It is also packed with ingredients to help boost your metabolism and keep you full longer. This kimbap recipe is from Qi Alchemy's blog post, "Healthy Kimbap Recipe."

SERVES 4

MULTIGRAIN RICE
1½ cups (252 g) uncooked multigrain rice, soaked for at least 3 hours
3 cups (700 ml) water
10 sesame leaves, julienned
2 tablespoons (28 ml) sesame oil
Salt

FILLING
2 eggs
Salt and black pepper
15 ounces (425 g) spinach
2 teaspoons soy sauce
2 teaspoons sesame oil
2 teaspoons sesame seeds
1 clove garlic, finely minced
1 cucumber
1 medium carrot
6 ounces (170 g) extra-firm tofu
1 can (5 ounces, or 140 g) tuna, drained

ASSEMBLY
3 sheets kim (dried laver seaweed), roasted slightly

1. Rice Preparation: Prepare rice by rinsing it with water until the water runs clear. Usually the water becomes clear after 5 to 7 rinses. Then, add the water and cook over medium-high heat for 7 to 10 minutes or until at a rolling boil. Stir the rice and make sure to scrape the bottom so the rice does not burn. Cover and lower to a simmer. Continue to cook for 12 to 15 minutes until the rice turns fluffy and is thoroughly cooked. Transfer the rice to a heatproof bowl and gently fold in the sesame oil and sesame leaves. Season with salt to taste.

2. Filling Preparation: Add a thin layer of cooking oil to a medium-sized pan and heat over medium heat. Beat the eggs with a little salt and pepper and add the eggs to the pan. Once the bottom is set, flip the egg over and cook all the way through. Transfer the eggs to a cutting board and cut into long strips.

3. Bring a saucepan of salted water to a boil and blanch the spinach for 30 seconds until softened. Drain and quickly rinse the spinach with cold water to preserve the color and nutrients. Gently squeeze the spinach to remove excess water. In a bowl, season the spinach with soy sauce, sesame oil, sesame seeds, and garlic. This is also a great side dish to make in bulk and eat with rice along with other pickled vegetables.

4. Slice the cucumber and discard the seeds. Then, slice it into long sticks. Julienne the carrot or cut it into ⅓-inch (8 mm) strips. Blanch the carrots in salted water until softened. Drain and then remove the excess water.

5. Remove any excess moisture from the tofu with a paper towel. Slice it into 4 pieces. Lightly sprinkle the tofu with salt. Heat a large frying pan with a little cooking oil over medium-high heat. Fry the tofu slices for 1 to 2 minutes or until all sides are golden brown.

6. Remove any excess liquid from the tuna with a paper towel.

7. Assembling the roll: Cover a bamboo rolling mat with plastic wrap to keep it clean. If you do not have a bamboo mat handy, you can use a clean kitchen towel. Place a sheet of the seaweed on the bamboo rolling mat, shiny-side down. Spread about ¾ cup (126 g) of rice on the seaweed, leaving a 1-inch (2.5 cm) edge at the top. Carefully place each filling in the center of the roll.

8. Using the bamboo mat, roll over the filling so that you reach the other end of the rice. Using firm pressure, keep rolling and tucking. Remove from the mat and set the kimbap aside with the seam-side down. Repeat two more times with the remaining ingredients. Brush the finished rolls with sesame oil.

9. Cut each roll into 6 to 8 pieces using a sharp knife. Wiping the knife with a damp paper towel between each slice will prevent the rice from sticking.

—

I delight in the spectrum of colorful foods—a festival of lights.

NOTES: Rather than white rice, I highly recommend consuming multigrain rice because whole-grain rice varieties contain less sugar and are beneficial in reducing heart disease and type 2 diabetes as well as obesity. Multigrain rice also contains many nutrients, fiber, and essential minerals such as magnesium, copper, zinc, and iron.

Tofu, which is made out of bean curd, has vitamins and minerals such as iron, calcium, potassium, magnesium, copper, zinc, and vitamin B_1. It helps lower cholesterol and is a great source of protein. Seaweed, a sea vegetable for ocean life, grows along the south coast of the Korean peninsula and is harvested in the winter and early spring. Seaweed is rich in iodine, a mineral essential for our metabolism and healthy thyroid function. Its high potassium and vitamin B_{12} content helps lower blood pressure and risk of heart disease and prevents cancer.

NUTRITION NOTES: Sesame leaves are rich in vitamins A, C, and B_2, minerals, calcium, iron, potassium, and omega-3 fatty acids. They are also high in fiber and help reduce inflammation.

THE POWER OF FIVE AND THIRD TASTE

When we deeply appreciate the taste of our food, we savor and feel our senses spark with different emotions. Imagine yourself near a firepit roasting deodeok root (bellflower root) seasoned with Korean red pepper flakes and placed on top of a roll of kimbap. While the root is roasted, feelings of joy or sorrow may come out depending on your constitution. The memories that fire brings to you may bring tears of joy, sorrow, or maybe peace.

Once the deodeok is roasted and ready to be eaten, we place it on top of our kimbap roll of seasoned herbs and vegetables. We close our eyes and smell the flavors and warmth near our faces. When we open our eyes and mouth and take a bite, the taste of the spicy root hits our lungs and then our large intestine.

The colorful vegetables and protein penetrate the spectrum of five cardinal colors, obagsaek, that shapes everything in our microcosmic body. This is the third taste, and we will explore it in the following chapters. One bite should be experienced in such a profound way that we will always remember where the root was from or how it was made for us.

THIRD TASTE REFLECTION

As we discover our third taste, take out a journal and write how the taste made you feel or what memories you thought of. Feelings of joy, sadness, anger, or delight may occur. There may be times when we lose our appetite and the foods we eat taste bland.

Ask yourself, "What is going on internally that is numbing my taste buds? How am I feeling these days? Am I ignoring or repressing certain feelings or emotions that I haven't addressed? Am I feeling off-balance? How is my health these days?"

Observing the changes that are happening in our lives can be a factor in being able to savor the taste of our foods. When we are in an optimal state and our Qi is in balance, joy and gratitude is felt in every bite.

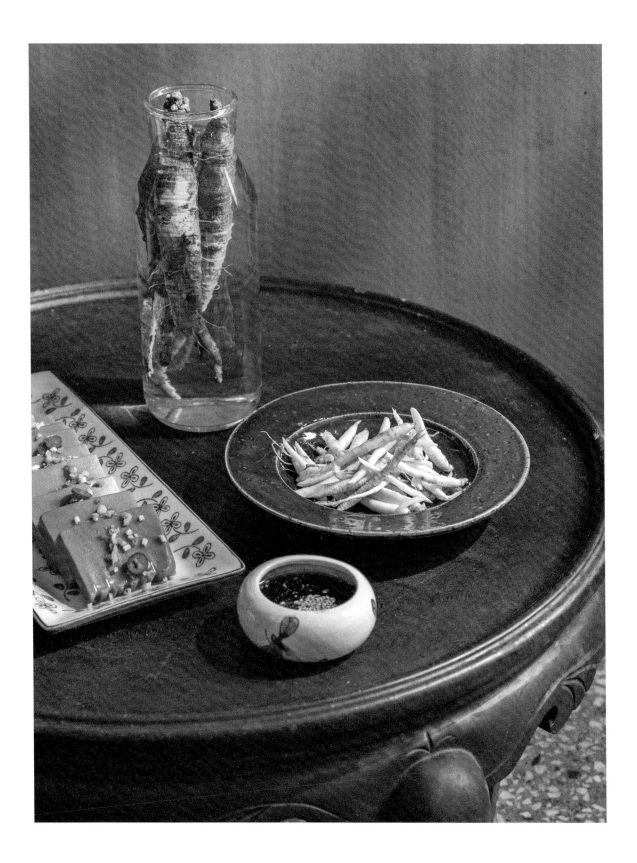

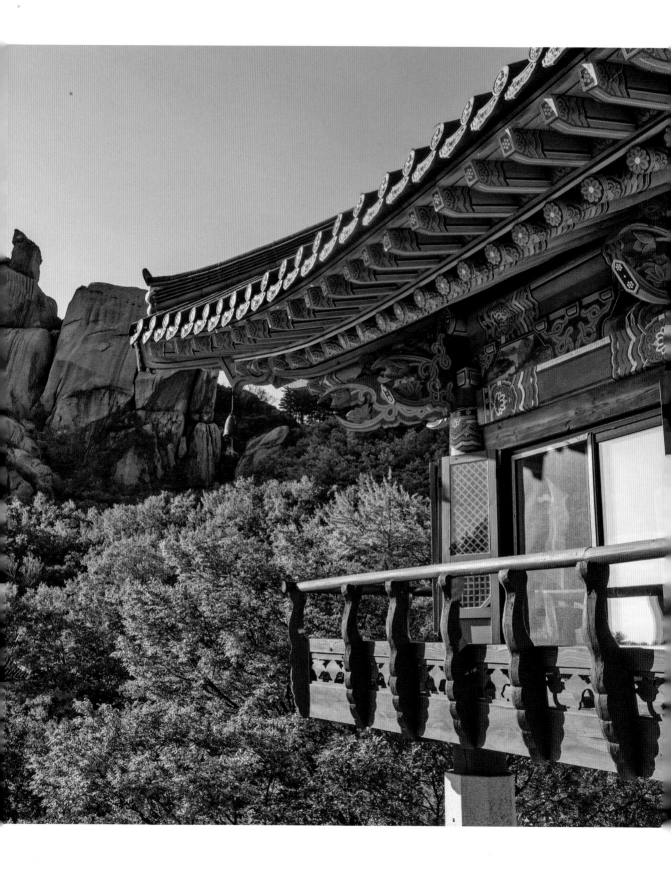

2 THE MEANING OF QI ALCHEMY

기 연금술 [gi yeongeumsul]

Flow like a river
Dream like a cloud
The river and sea are one
The sun and moon remain the same
So dance to the rhythm of the wind as ashes of life and death are one
On the mountaintop, we see clearly the beauty and splendor of the vital life force
A living sun shining inside us

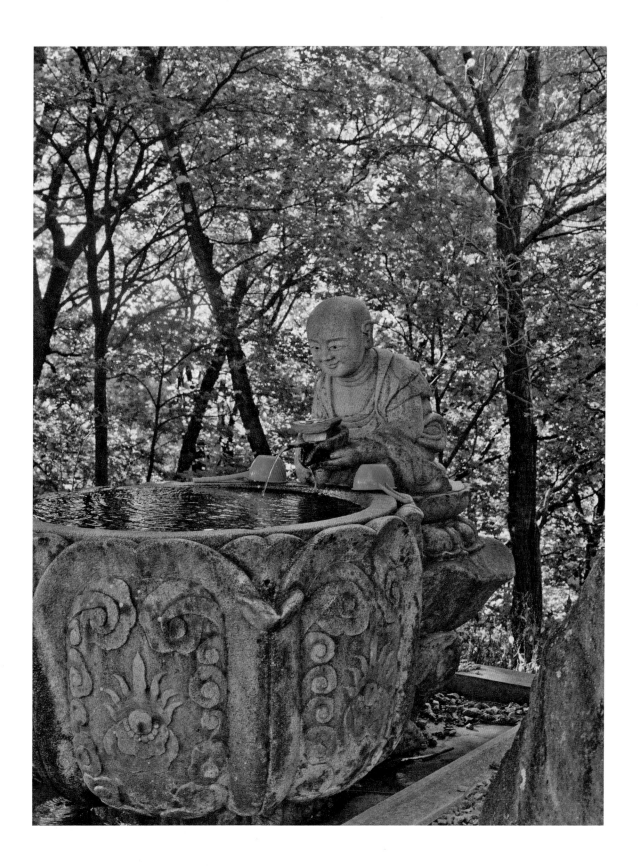

VITAL LIFE FORCE, QI

Qi is our vital life force, and the flow of this energy around and through us constantly needs to balance. Understanding our personal rhythm and flow of Qi is essential for stable equilibrium and longevity, and once we master our personal flow of Qi, we become healing herbalists for others.

Similar to pronouncing herb with or without the "h" [erb], Qi is pronounced differently depending on the geographical region in Asia. In China, it is pronounced with a "c" like *chi*, and in Korea, it is pronounced with a "k" like *key*. When you hear the word, be mindful that it has the same meaning and is simply pronounced differently.

The godfather of Korean medicine, Heo Jun wrote *Dongui Bogam*, one of the most significant texts that distinguished the practice of Korean medicine from traditional Eastern medicine. It is one of the classics of Eastern medicine. In his book, he writes:

> One the most precious living things in the universe is mankind. Our round head resembles heaven, and our flat foot resembles earth. We have four limbs as the universe has four seasons. We have five viscera as the universe has five phases. We have twelve meridians as the universe has twelve hours. Man has twenty-four acupoints as the universe has twenty-four Qi.
>
> We have 365 joints as the universe has 365 divisions. We have 2 eyes as the universe has the sun and the moon. We sleep and wake as the universe has day and night. We have happiness and anger as the universe has thunder and lightning, and we have tears and nasal discharge as the universe has rain and dew. We have cold and heat as the universe has yin and yang, and we have blood vessels as the universe has spring water. We have hair growing as the universe has grass and trees growing, and we have teeth as the universe has metals and rocks.

As a child, my grandma would use her hands to cure me. Whenever I had a headache, Grandma would press the tip of my middle finger and my headache would go away. Whenever I had a stomachache, she would press between my index finger and thumb and my stomach pain would disappear. I'm not sure what magical healing powers Grandma had, but I know that understanding our body constitution brings us more consciousness.

We each have a mini cosmos and components of the universe in us. Herbs also have their own life force, their own Qi. Our environment, the four seasons, acupuncture points, they all share a united frequency that exists in us. So, whenever we tilt our heads up to look at the clouds, remember that heaven is round, and when our feet touch the soil, we are feeling the flatness of earth. When we are joyful in spirit or our eyes are full of tears, the universe has wind and rain.

Sources of Qi

We go through different layers in life, and we experience three sources of Qi during our lifetime. When we were newborns, our scent was distinct—our blood was pure and flowing. We had a new lens on the world and were in a state of wonder. Everything is fresh, and on a physical level, our **inherited source** is transmitted to us from our parents.

As we spend more time in the world and become independent, our second source is the **foods we eat** to keep our bodies alive and thriving. The nutrients that we receive from our meals give us fuel to sustain a healthy lifestyle. Everyone's eating habits are different, and it is crucial to learn about the nutritious foods that affect our health and longevity. Unfortunately, our food and education system has failed to inform us about nutrition, and those who have been fortunate to grow up with healthy eating habits have the advantage of knowing what nutritious foods to eat.

As herbalists, it is our responsibility to learn the fundamentals of nutrition and to educate others on how simple herbs can be used for everyday cooking. It is never too late to change our eating habits, especially in our thirties and forties while our taste buds continue to develop. It may be hard at first, but I believe we all have the courage to change if we really want to make a lasting difference in our lives.

Many people have asked for my support in helping them shift their lifestyle and eating habits. As a first step, I always ask how they remember their younger self:

- What were you usually eating when you were five years old?
- How did food make you feel when you were a child?
- Did you cook with your family or eat out most of the time?
- Did your diet change as a teenager?
- Are there any foods that you really crave during certain moments or special occasions?
- What do you normally eat as an adult?

They say infants have around thirty thousand taste buds, and by the time we hit adulthood, only one-third of our taste buds remain. The evolution of our food is changing constantly as our food industry is adding GMOs and alternative sweeteners and emulsifiers. Pause and reflect on the changes that we've made in our eating habits and how this affects your well-being.

Lastly, the **air we breathe** gives us the oxygen for our hearts to beat. We do not really think enough about the quality of air we breathe, but long-term exposure to poor air quality can impact our longevity. There are numerous studies on the exposure to ozone and how it can inflame and irritate the lining of the respiratory system, causing conditions such as asthma and impaired breathing. As the years go by, small particles can build up internally and affect our respiratory system. There are ways that we can control our indoor air quality by using HEPA filters and nontoxic paint. One of my favorite ways to breathe outdoor air is standing by the ocean—the fresh, invigorating air blowing onto the shore from the sea feels different from static air by the road.

All three sources are part of Qi and are in constant motion. We ascend, descend, enter, and leave. As you begin your journey, I encourage you to start by increasing your awareness. Write down everything you are eating and drinking

for seven days. From this exercise, you will see the fresh and processed foods that you are consuming on a regular basis. This awareness is the first step to making gradual change. For those who are mindfully eating fresh nutritious foods, I encourage you to share your knowledge with others. Many people simply may not know much about nutrients in their foods. For your own health, continue to pay attention to what you eat and consume fermented foods and soups frequently if you are not already doing so.

THE VINEGAR TASTERS

Long ago, the founding fathers of Eastern philosophy—Taoism, Buddhism, and Confucianism—circled around a vat full of vinegar that represented the essence of life. Each of the founding fathers dipped their finger and tasted the vinegar, and each teacher had a different expression and perspective.

Confucianism

A sour taste. The vinegar tasted sour to Confucius as modern life has strayed from the sacred rituals and traditions of the past. The bridge between heaven and earth is ancestral and cultural heritage, and if morality declines, society has drifted away from the Way of Heaven. Confucius believed that ancestral rituals create order, which leads to the right results.

The basis of Confucianism is to live virtuously and bring peace and order to the world. Loyalty and respect to family, especially to our elders and ancestors, is important as it is key to the circle of life. Without our ancestors, mothers, and fathers, we would not exist in this world. Confucianism is social rituals, but beyond that, it also focuses on education and humanness in building character.

Confucianism had a major impact in shaping Korean culture, and its fundamental practice is living peacefully in the world. Korean culture places emphasis on Confucian ideology along with Buddhism and Taoism.

Words of Wisdom from Confucius

"Study the past if you want to define the future."

"Everything has beauty but not everyone sees it."

"Life is really simple, but we insist on making it complicated."

"Wisdom, compassion, and courage are the three universally recognized moral qualities of men."

"It does not matter how slowly you go as long as you do not stop."

"It is easy to hate and it is difficult to love. This is how the whole scheme of things works. All good things are difficult to achieve, and bad things are very easy to get."

Buddhism

Bitter as life. Buddha's taste of the vinegar was embittered as he viewed life as full of suffering and the modern world as deceitful. The worldly illusions that motivate people eventually lead to pain. Society's obsession with the pursuit of personal accomplishment and materialism brings bitterness and suffering. In Korea, shamanism influenced Buddhism throughout the centuries where monks performed shamanistic rituals in dance and music. Shamanism was the indigenous religion, and many shamans helped grow the Buddhist religion. The locations in the mountains where they held ceremonies later became the sites where Buddhist temples were built. Usually in Korea, there is a mountain god shrine next to the temple for rituals and to pay respect. There are at least one hundred thousand practicing shamans in Korea, and the majority of shamans are women.

The philosophy of Buddhism focuses on how one can improve oneself to achieve enlightenment and attain the state of nirvana. The path to enlightenment could be found by living in simplicity and moderation. The fundamental practice is how to live with yourself. Buddhism has played an important role in Korean history for about 1,600 years, and it remains one of the major religions in South Korea today.

Buddhist Sayings

"If you are quiet enough, you will hear the flow of the universe. You will feel its rhythm. Go with this flow. Happiness lies ahead. Meditation is key."

"Every morning we are born again. What we do today is what matters most."

"The secret of health for both mind and body is not to mourn for the past, nor to worry about the future, but to live the present moment wisely and earnestly."

"As a water bead on a lotus leaf, as water on a red lily, does not adhere, so the sage does not adhere to the seen, the heard, or the sensed."

"She who knows life flows, feels no wear or tear, needs no mending or repair."

"Health is the greatest gift, contentment the greatest wealth, faithfulness the best relationship."

Taoism

Sweet vinegar. Lao Tzu, the father of Taoism, tasted sweetness, which was a reflection of his philosophy of the world as harmonious in its natural state. Taoists believe that there is a constant state of flow and harmony between heaven and earth. As humans are advancing with technology and interfering with the natural state of the world, more distance and friction is caused between humanity and the harmony of the universe.

Taoism is based on how one can become aligned with nature and the cosmos as well as being in touch with our real selves. Instead of spending a great deal of time worrying about who we ought to become, we should take the time to be who we already are at heart. The fundamental practice is how to live in one with nature.

Words of Wisdom from Lao Tzu

"Watch your thoughts, they become your words; watch your words, they become your actions; watch your actions, they become your habits; watch your habits, they become

your character; watch your character, it becomes your destiny."

"Life is a series of natural and spontaneous changes. Don't resist them; that only creates sorrow. Let reality be reality."

"Simplicity, patience, compassion. These three are your greatest treasures."

"Let things flow naturally forward in whatever way they like."

"When I let go of what I am, I become what I might be."

"Everything under heaven is a sacred vessel and cannot be controlled. Trying to control leads to ruin. Trying to grasp, we lose. Allow your life to unfold naturally. Know that it too is a vessel of perfection. Just as you breathe in and breathe out, there is a time for being ahead and a time for being behind; a time for being in motion and a time for being at rest; a time for being vigorous and a time for being exhausted; a time for being safe and a time for being in danger."

"Be careful what you water your dreams with. Water them with worry and fear and you will produce weeds that choke the life from your dream. Water them with optimism and solutions and you will cultivate success. Always be on the lookout for ways to turn a problem into an opportunity for success. Always be on the lookout for ways to nurture your dream."

Lessons from the Three Vinegar Tasters

Life circumstances teach us lessons that may be painful or enlightening—it's really a matter of perspective and our decision to seek clarity in our future.

As the vinegar tasters experience the sourness or bitterness of life, we can stay in a place of anger or resentment or simply appreciate what the universe has to offer. Openness, adaptability, and appreciation to the lessons in life will bring sweetness and harmony into our lives.

Vinegars in Our Herbal Apothecary

식초 [sikcho]

Vinegar is an essential liquid that we use in everyday culinary arts as well as for fermenting and pickling foods. Vinegars in Asia are often less acidic and usually mixed with a fermented herb, vegetable, or fruit. Some vinegars to add to our herbal apothecary include brown rice vinegar, wolfberry (goji berry) vinegar, persimmon vinegar, barley vinegar, and mugwort vinegar.

Umma loved all types of vinegar. She would buy gallons of vinegar from big-box stores and make pickled radish, cabbage, cucumbers, mustard greens, and perilla leaves. The smell of vinegar is pungent, sour, or bitter, and she would say that smell and taste are just basic senses. The third sense that we must use to taste is *shewonhan mat* (시원한 맛). This third taste is a nourishing taste that you feel when you eat and digest—the ultimate sensation through our tongue, stomach, and intestines during the digestive process. The balance of temperature, acidity, sweetness, saltiness, or sour concentration of foods brings the unique sensation of different herbal blends with vinegars.

Brown Rice Vinegar

Rice vinegar is derived from fermented rice, and its active ingredients and compounds have many health benefits such as improving the immune system, promoting digestion, boosting energy, and enhancing skin care. It is also a great liver tonic because of its detoxifying properties. In addition to its many health benefits, brown rice vinegar contains amino acids that help the body fight fatigue.

Wolfberry Vinegar

Antioxidant-rich wolfberries or goji berries help protect eye health, increase blood production, and improve memory. An antioxidant in goji berries, zeaxanthin, helps stabilize free radicals and oxidative stress. It also stabilizes blood sugar levels and provides immune support. Studies have shown that wolfberry increases white blood

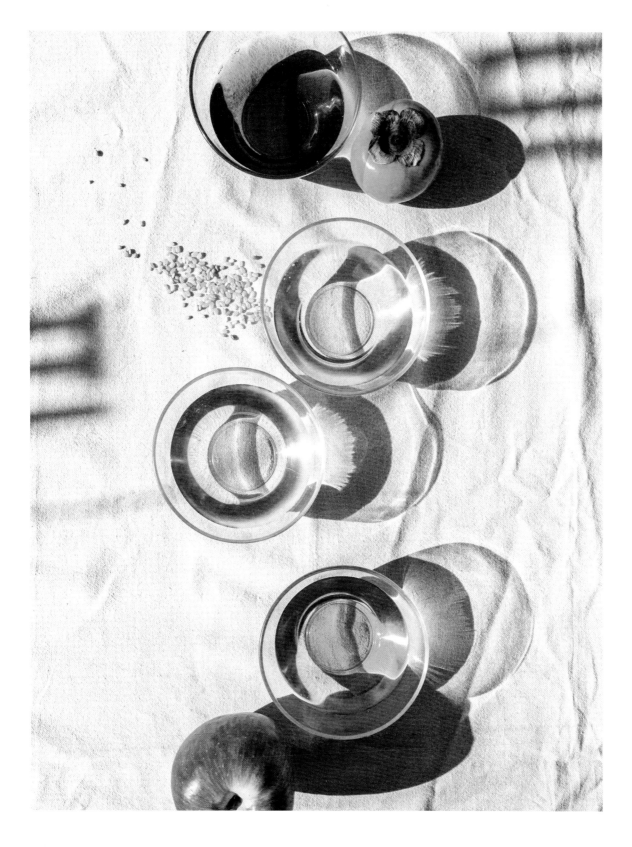

cell production when consumed on a regular basis. This vinegar is used to enhance the flavor of fish, salads, white meats, and steamed vegetables.

Persimmon Vinegar

Similar to having apple cider vinegar as an essential pantry staple, Koreans also store persimmon vinegar. The unique flavor has smooth-tasting notes of sweet and sour. A tablespoon (15 ml) of persimmon vinegar a day has tremendous health benefits that support your heart, liver, skin, and digestion. Persimmon has a sweet honey flavor, contains phytonutrients, and is rich in vitamins A, C, and K. It also has a high fiber and mineral content.

Barley Vinegar

The malted germinating grains of barley go through a double fermentation process where the grains are malted and brewed into ale. Then, the second fermentation process turns the ale into vinegar where it is aged. Barley has many beneficial nutrients such as fiber and beta-glucans that help with cholesterol levels and magnesium that may prevent diabetes. Rich in vitamins, minerals, and plant compounds, barley, which should be a regular grain in our diet, offers protection from chronic disease.

Mugwort Vinegar

Mugwort vinegar is a perfect cleansing tonic for the fall. Mugwort promotes blood circulation, aids digestion, and protects the liver. When making your own mugwort vinegar, take the opportunity to reflect as part of the overall experience. Remember the vinegar tasters and each of their philosophies on life. Which philosophy do you lean toward more? If there is a particular philosophy that draws you, I encourage you to be curious and learn more about Taoism, Buddhism, or Confucianism or all three. Exploring and understanding more about different cultures will expand your awareness to native herbs and how the East practices herbalism.

As the founding fathers of Taoism, Buddhism, and Confucianism once tasted vinegar in their own way, we too should taste the different notes of various vinegars available to us and meditate on how we perceive life. If life is currently bitter or sour, how can we make it a bit sweeter? If life is too sweet, how can we balance it with bitter or sour notes? Through simple and essential ingredients such as vinegar, we can learn the essence of life.

Time and time again, we cleanse and trust
Cleanse and trust
We stretch out our hands as we feel the wind between our fingers
We close our eyes as the sun beams on our face
We clap and bow to Mother Nature as she oversees all things
So we cleanse and trust
Cleanse and trust
Time and time again

MUGWORT PERSIMMON VINEGAR

식초에 절인 양배추 [sigcho-e jeol-in yangbaechu]

MAKES 1 PINT (473 ML)

1½ cups (60 g) chopped
fresh mugwort leaves
and stems or ¾ cup
(24 g) dried mugwort
10 to 12 ounces (285 to
355 ml) persimmon
vinegar

Adding an earthy herbal-flavored vinegar enhances the taste of rooted vegetables and meat dishes. Mugwort is known to cleanse and aid digestion as well as strengthen the immune system.

1. Place the mugwort in a clean and sanitized 16-ounce (473 ml) mason jar. Pour persimmon vinegar over the herbs to cover them completely until the liquid reaches to nearly the top of the mason jar.

2. Stir with a chopstick to remove any air bubbles. Place a sheet of wax paper or cheesecloth over the top of the mason jar. This prevents the vinegar from corroding the lid. Cap tightly with the lid. Let it steep for at least 6 weeks in a cool, dark place. Shake the medicine each time you see it.

3. When the mugwort is ready, strain out the herbs through a fine-mesh sieve. Discard the plant material and decant the remaining liquid in a dark-colored glass bottle and label it with the ingredients and when it was made. Take this medicine by consuming 1 tablespoon (15 ml) a day.

—

Sour moments in life bring a new rebirth. The moment I accept myself as I am, all the sour burdens will disappear and will become sweet like persimmon.

PICKLED CABBAGE AND
CITRON HONEY–VINEGAR DRESSING

유자 꿀 식초 드레싱 [yuja kkul sigcho deulesing]

SERVES 4

PICKLED CABBAGE
½ head leafy green or
purple cabbage
2 cups (475 ml) white or
brown rice vinegar
1 cup (225 g) packed
brown sugar
1 teaspoon salt

**CITRON HONEY–
VINEGAR DRESSING**
1 tablespoon (20 g) citron
honey (substitute any
organic honey)
Lemon juice, to taste
3 tablespoons (45 ml)
olive oil
1 tablespoon (15 ml)
persimmon vinegar

Cabbage is part of the Brassica oleracea family. For this recipe, pickled cabbage is paired with a simple herbal dressing. The sweet flavor is refreshing and universal for everyone to enjoy. These components are always stocked in my fridge. If you love the taste, make a mason jar full of the dressing by multiplying the recipe by ten.

1. To make the cabbage: Cut and quarter the cabbage into slices. Then, fully pack the sliced cabbage into a 16-ounce (475 ml) mason jar. Combine the vinegar, brown sugar, and salt. Pour the vinegar mixture into the mason jar until the cabbage is fully covered with the liquid.

2. To make the dressing: Combine the citron honey, lemon juice, olive oil, and persimmon vinegar in a bowl. Whisk together to make a smooth dressing.

—

Go within your heart, pick three words, then eat.

Courage	Gratitude	Integrity
Health	Joy	Openness
Peace	Truth	Abundance
Forgiveness	Passion	Surrender

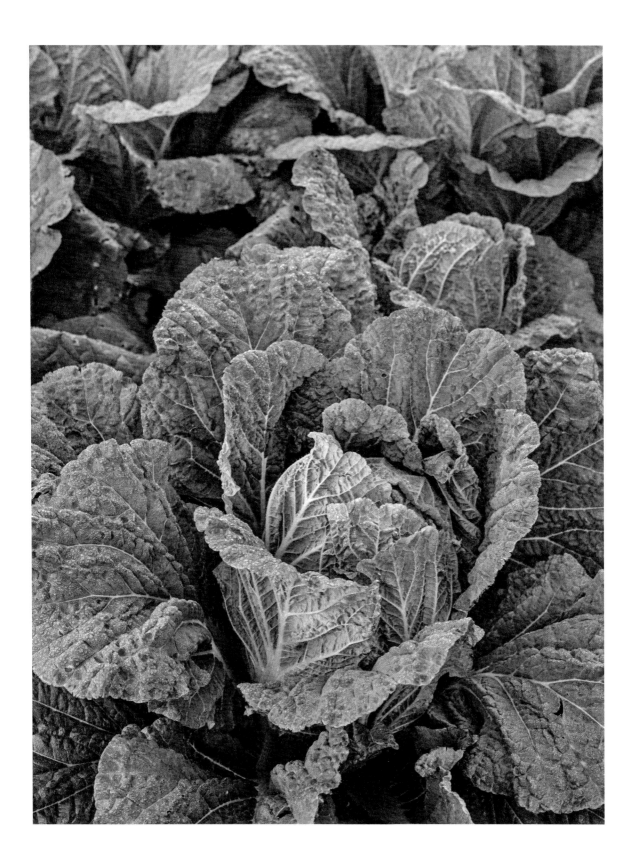

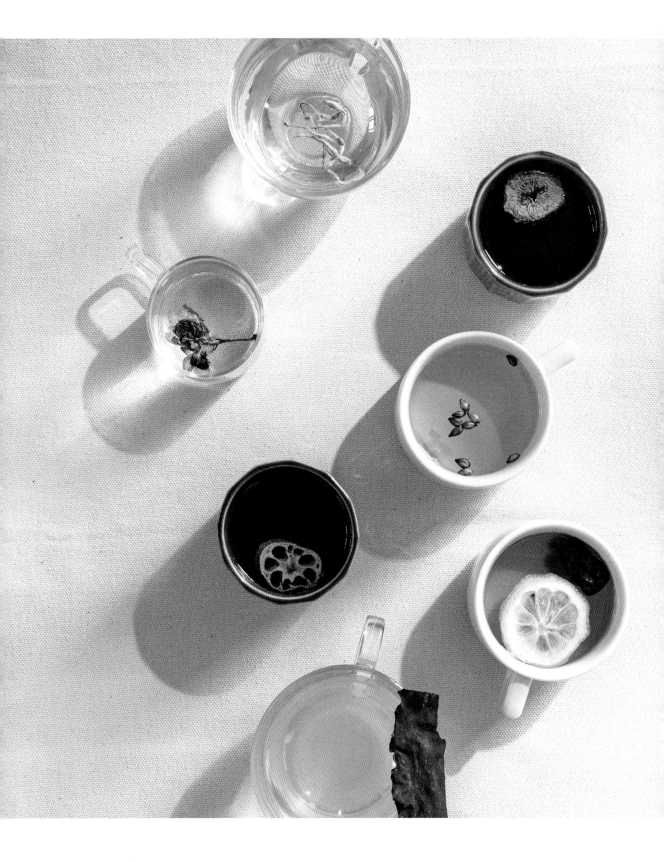

3 | CONSTITUTIONAL MEDICINE AND HERBAL ESSENTIALS

사상의학 [sasang-uihag]

Compass of Our Hearts
North or South
East or West
Treading carefully as we decide which way is best
Straight and narrow
Circles and zigzags
We want clarity and safety to bring us peace
The compass of our hearts is in Mother Nature
So whatever path we take
At the end,
It leads us to the same way.

CONSTITUTIONAL MEDICINE

Similar to Ayurveda in India, Korea has a system of holistic medicine based on a person's typological constitution called the Sasang constitution. This includes psychological, social, and physical characteristics. *Sasang* literally means "four symbols," and the four symbols are the four body types that we will explore in this chapter.

The main philosophical basis for Sasang is that human nature and interpersonal relationships are rooted in Confucian foundations, whereas traditional Chinese medicine is based on Taoist principles. The founding medical doctor and scholar, Yi Je-ma, devoted his life to studying longevity and life preservation in Eastern medicine and developed the Sasang constitution.

Each person is born with varying energetic, emotional, and physical strengths and weaknesses depending on our body type. Our natural constitution is different, and disease should be treated differently depending on our biophysical traits.

In Sasang theory, humans have two features: the mind and the body. The mind is the same as the heart, and it is divided into four emotions: sorrow, anger, joy, and pleasure. The body is divided into organ systems: the lung, liver, pancreas, and kidney. Each person has stronger and weaker energetic organs, and according to Sasang medicine, the difference in energetic strength is what promotes a balanced Qi. The mind-heart governs the entire body, and four body types are based on a person's biopsychosocial traits as well as yin-yang theory.

GREATER YIN

태음 [Tae Eum]

People of the Tae Eum constitution have strong liver energy and weak lungs. They tend to be thoughtful and slow as well as deliberate. The emotional effect to the liver is complacency while the lungs link to sorrow. They generally have warm central energy. Roughly 30 percent of the population is Tae Eum.

BODY SHAPE: thick waist and weak nape of the neck, round face, long legs

CHARACTERISTICS: pragmatic, resilient, humorous, reflective, cautious, desire for joy, reserved

PHYSICAL: strong absorption of food and fat tissue, tendency to gain weight easily

NATURE: joy

HERBS TO USE: ginkgo nuts, acorn, pine nuts, Job's tears, sesame seeds, turmeric, bean sprouts, chestnuts, arrowroot, lotus root, dandelion greens, bamboo shoots

HERBAL TEAS TO DRINK: dandelion, chamomile, green tea, white tea

FIVE FUSION TEA

파이브 퓨전 티 [paibeu pyujeon ti]

MAKES 3½ CUPS (820 ML) OF TEA

1 piece fresh ginger,
  1-inch (2.5 cm)
15 cloves garlic
7 jujubes
7 ginkgo nuts
7 chestnuts, peeled
7 cups (1.6 L) water
Honey, to taste
Pine nuts or sliced
  jujubes, for garnish

For people with Tae Eum constitution, this powerful fusion of garlic, ginger, ginkgo, jujube, and chestnut has healing properties that boost the immune system, relieve coughs, and lower cholesterol levels. It relieves constipation and improves virility. The Five Fusion Tea is also for people who have a weakened immune system from chronic illnesses, high cholesterol, and constipation.

1. Wash and drain the ginger, garlic, jujubes, ginkgo nuts, and chestnuts. Add them to a large saucepan over medium-high heat with the water. Bring to a boil.

2. Reduce the heat and simmer until reduced by half. Strain the tea through a fine-mesh sieve.

3. Serve the tea hot, sweetened with honey to taste and garnished with pine nuts or jujubes. Refrigerate any unused tea in an airtight container for up to 10 days.

—

We are all a part of the whole microbial diversity. Sip the diverse infusion.

℘

NOTE: The great thing about drinking herbal teas is that they rarely have any contraindicated side effects because of the light dose of herbs, and they are gentle to digest. Be mindful of how your body feels when drinking the tea. If it feels nourishing, feel free to drink it on a regular basis. If not, then hold off on drinking more and try other types of herbal teas.

LESSER YIN

소음 [So Eum]

People who are So Eum have very strong kidney energy and a weak pancreas. Often related to winter because of their cold central energy, they have a cold and damp system. Their energy is stagnant because coldness starts to increase after the solstice. To balance their bodies, they need a great amount of warmth. People with So Eum body types should avoid damp, wet foods as well as moist and humid environments. Vegetarian and vegan diets are not suitable for them unless their daily meals are very hot and spicy. The majority of the population (about 40 percent) is So Eum.

BODY SHAPE: developed hips and small chest, narrow shoulders

CHARACTERISTICS: organized, logical, calm, introverted, persistent, egocentric, quiet

PHYSICAL: stronger lower body than upper body and often short and thin, deep-set eyes

NATURE: pleasure

HERBS TO USE: ginseng, clementine or tangerine peel, cinnamon, astragalus, ginger, horseradish, mustard seeds, rosemary, fennel, chives, anise

HERBAL TEAS TO DRINK: ginger, cinnamon, jujube, ginseng, clove, licorice, citrus teas

CITRUS HERB TEA

시트러스 허브 티 [siteuleoseu heobeu ti]

MAKES 5 CUPS (1.2 L) OF TEA

1 medium-sized ginseng
¼ cup (23 g) wolfberry (goji berry)
¼ cup (24 g) clementine peel
10 cups (2.4 L) water
Honey, for serving

The combination of ginseng, wolfberry (goji berry), and clementine is a great blend for So Eum constitution. It boosts energy and stamina as well as strengthens the immune system. It also has antiaging properties. This tea helps stimulate appetite after having been sick or recovering from surgery. Citrus Herb Tea is also good for people with a weak immune system who need to increase their stamina and appetite.

1. Thoroughly wash the ginseng, wolfberry, and clementine peel. Peel the ginseng skin and cut the ginseng root into small slices. Add all the ingredients to a medium-sized pan over medium-high heat with the water. Bring to a boil.

2. Reduce the heat and simmer until the liquid is reduced by half. Strain through a fine-mesh sieve and then cool the liquid in the refrigerator for at least 1 hour or overnight.

3. Drink hot or cold depending on whether you run hot or cold: Drink hot tea if you run colder, and vice versa. Serve with a teaspoon (20 g) of honey for sweetness.

—

Create a clear vision for my life that allows me to have all I want. Never settle for only part of a possibility.

NOTE: You can rebrew this tea right away by adding more water to further extract the healing properties from the ingredients.

GREATER YANG

태양 [Tae Yang]

Tae Yang people have strong lung energy and a weak liver. Therefore, they should consume foods that strengthen the liver and avoid foods that strengthen the lung to achieve a balanced Qi. Their central energy is hot, so they need to avoid foods and herbs that are warming in nature. A very small percentage of the population (about 1 percent) is this body type.

BODY SHAPE: slender waist and developed naped neck, large torso

CHARACTERISTICS: creative, progressive, charismatic, heroic, active, outgoing, easily excited

PHYSICAL: strongly developed neck and head, small waistline, large face, and shiny eyes

NATURE: sorrow

HERBS TO USE: black sesame seeds, quince extract, grape root extract, black currant, bitter gourd, persimmon, buckwheat

HERBAL TEAS TO DRINK: pine needle, quince tea, persimmon leaf tea

FERMENTED PINE NEEDLE TEA

솔잎차 [sol-ipcha]

MAKES 4 CUPS (946 ML) OF TEA

16 ounces (455 g) Korean red pine needles or Eastern white pine needles (found in the US)
4 cups (946 ml) water
16 ounces (455 g) brown sugar, or more if needed

Pine needles are harvested in the winter from ten- to twenty-year-old trees. Older pine needles compared with young needles contain more tannins and tend to taste bitter, so try to harvest young pine needles for a smoother taste. Taoist teachers consumed pine needle tea because they believed it extended their longevity. Pine needles have detoxifying and antiaging properties and have abundant health benefits with high levels of vitamins A, B, and C. The needles have five times the concentration of vitamin C found in lemons. This tea is great for throat, sinus, and lung health, and it is a decongestant and expectorant.

1. Thoroughly clean the pine needles in water to remove the sticky resin. Infuse the dried pine needles in the water over low heat for 10 minutes and then strain.

2. Weigh the pine needles and add the same amount of sugar as the weight of the pine needles into a 32-ounce (946 ml) mason jar. Fill the mason jar with water until the pine needles are fully submerged.

3. Ferment the pine needle concentrate for at least 3 to 6 months in a closed, dark place. Once it is fully fermented, add a tablespoon (15 ml) of the concentrate in a cup (235 ml) of hot or cold water and enjoy it as a tea!

—

An anchor to the ground, let me adapt to the extremities of life like the pine tree.

LESSER YANG

소양 [So Yang]

So Yang people have strong pancreas energy and weaker kidneys. The summer season represents their constitution because of their hot and dry systems and rising internal heat. They need to avoid anything that increases heat and dryness and that strengthens the stomach and spleen. They thrive on foods that are cooling and moistening in nature. About 30 percent of the population is So Yang.

BODY SHAPE: developed chest, small hips

CHARACTERISTICS: extroverted, social, moody, sacrificing, easily bored, hot-tempered, righteous

PHYSICAL: weaker lower body, thin, and prone to adrenal fatigue

NATURE: anger

HERBS TO USE: burdock, mung beans, seaweed, wolfberry (goji berry), ginger extract, barley, soy beans, taro root, rehmannia

HERBAL TEAS TO DRINK: mint, jasmine, barley, peppermint

M3 (MINERAL MARINE MOISTURE) TEA

해초차 [haecho]

MAKES 4 CUPS (946 ML) OF TEA

¼ cup (58 g) dashi
3 to 5 cups (700 ml to 1.2 L) water
Salt, to taste (optional)

We quench our thirst by drinking minerals from the sea. This M3 Tea will keep you hydrated and help retain moisture for your skin.

1. Wipe the dashi with a clean damp cloth or paper towel. Cut the dashi into small pieces.

2. In a small pan, boil the water over medium-high heat. Add the dashi to the boiling water, remove the pan from the stove, and let the dashi infuse for 5 minutes.

3. Strain through a fine-mesh strainer. Add salt if desired and drink hot.

—

We pray and drink dashi. Prayer brings peace. Prayer for your loved ones brings comfort and joy.

Dashi and Seaweed

If we see our future in seaweed—woven strands and countless species of mineral marine life—we see a rich life. Seaweed and dashi are essential sea herbs that are a Korean pantry staple. They are rich in vitamins and minerals, including iron, iodine, and calcium. In Eastern medicine, dashi is used to treat high blood pressure and anemia. It increases the metabolism and is an energy booster. Both dashi and seaweed are great to help with fatigue and constipation.

Taking a Constitutional Approach

Discovering your Sasang constitution is an ever-evolving process. What we express outwardly may be only a small part of what we feel deep inside. Throughout the years, we also may develop traits that may not be associated with our body type. The matrix of our mind and body is complex, and there are layers of who we are on the inside that we may not show outwardly, and vice versa. Throughout the seasons of life, we are evolving and one with nature.

We are unique beings, and no one person is the same. Our external features, psychological characteristics, the equilibrium among internal organic functions, and our sensitivity to certain foods, herbs, and medicines all differ from person to person. But the process in which our bodily fluids consume and discharge food is the same. Taking a constitutional approach can minimize the risk of adverse reactions to herbs and our foods while increasing their efficacy. This helps give us what we need to prevent chronic disease.

The simplest way to begin to assess your body type is to relate to a shape: Is your body type a triangle, upside-down triangle, oval, rectangle, or hourglass? What is your waist size? Then, consider your characteristics: What is your personality like? Do you consider yourself an introvert or extrovert? When making decisions, do you tend to overthink or make decisions quickly? Do you consider yourself more of a logical or emotional person?

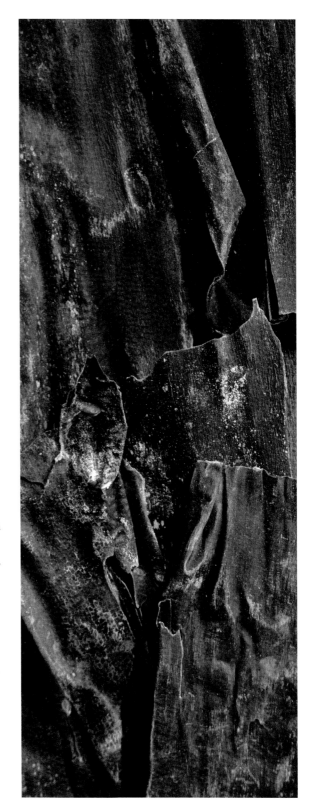

ESSENTIALS FOR YOUR KOREAN HERBAL APOTHECARY

As we begin building our Korean herbal apothecary, there are essential culinary and medicinal herbs that are foundational in making herbal remedies.

Sacred Rice

Rice is the symbol of life and prosperity. Twists of sacred rice straw are made when a child is born. The rice straw is braided, symbolizing purity and fertility. It is hung over the front gate of the newborn's home, announcing his or her birth and warding off evil forces. When a child is born into this world, the main object is keeping this little being safe. Twisting strands of rice straw to the left side is used for special rituals to have the supernatural ward off evil. It is a reminder for families to live carefully each day as the baby is highly sensitive to everything and needs to feel safe.

If the baby is a boy, charcoal, mulberry paper, and red peppers are twisted into the braid. Charcoal is used to burn all impurities and purify other materials. The mulberry paper strips are regarded as a mark of sacredness as Koreans regard the color of white paper as divine. The red peppers are a phallic symbol in Korea, and it is believed that evil spirits are scared of the color red. If the baby is a girl, charcoal, mulberry paper strips, and pine branches are twisted into the braid. The sharp needle leaves of a pine branch help repel evil, and the evergreen leaves are a symbol of fidelity.

The rope is hung for at least twenty-one days to forty-nine days announcing the birth of a new life and also symbolizing the blocking of evil energy from a new life. Then, the rope is burned at a clean place, letting Mother Nature know that the newborn's life is protected from evil forces and is ready to learn about the world.

Multigrain Rice

Korean multigrain rice is a healthy mixed-grain rice that includes grains and beans such as sorghum, millet, red or black beans, and even chickpeas. On the first full moon of the lunar calendar, we eat multigrain rice for breakfast, and we share the rice with our neighbors to receive a good harvest and fortune throughout the year.

The most common rice and grains infused in multigrain rice are as follows:

- Brown rice 현미 (hyun mi)
- Black rice 흑미 (heuk mi)
- Sweet rice 찹쌀 (chap ssal)
- Glutinous foxtail millet 차조 (cha jo)
- Proso millet 기장 (gi jang)
- Sorghum 수수 (susu)

CHOOSE HEALTHY RICE

A daily Korean meal is always served with rice, but not all rice is the same nutritionally. White rice has a high glycemic index, so avoid white rice if possible.

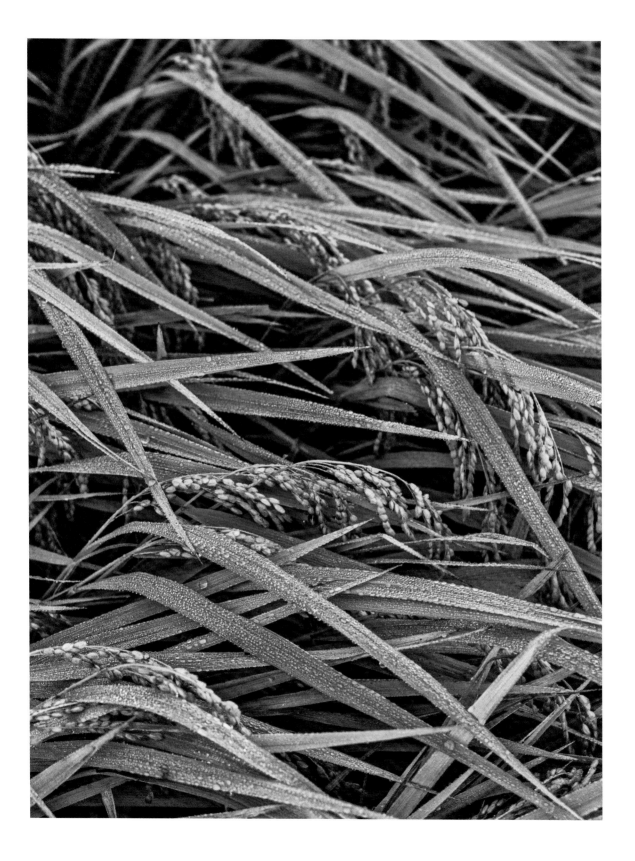

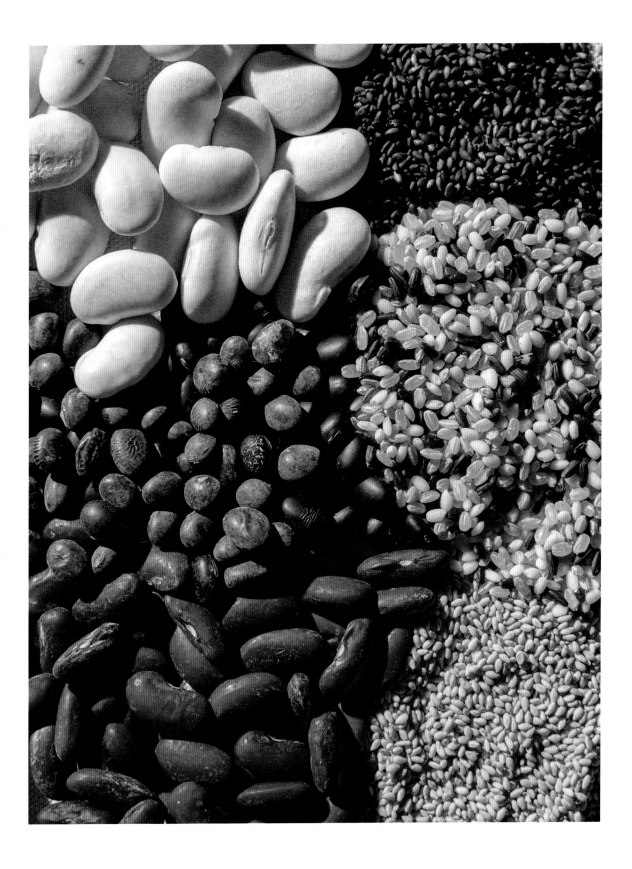

Some common beans mixed into the multigrain rice are as follows:

- Black beans 검은 콩 (geom-eun kong)
- Kidney beans 신장 콩 (shin-jang kong)
- Adzuki red beans 팥 (pat)
- Chickpeas 병아리콩 (byeong-ali kong)
- Lentils 렌틸 콩 (lentil kong)

Soak all dry beans and grains for at least six hours. Be sure to change the water at least three times or when the water becomes clear during the soaking process (except for regular short-grain rice and sweet rice) and then cook in a rice cooker. One cup (168 g) of rice will usually take about 17 to 18 minutes.

All grains and beans contain phytic acid, which is the main form of storage for phosphorus in seeds. It binds minerals in the intestinal tract and inhibits their absorption. Fermenting grains helps to predigest their proteins.

Flours of the Earth

밀가루 [milgalu]

From the ground, we produce flours of the earth. A wheat kernel is composed of three parts: the bran, germ, and endosperm. During the milling process, the parts are separated and recombined to produce different types of flour. Whole wheat flour contains all three parts of the kernel, whereas white flour is only ground endosperm. Noodles, rice cakes, and Korean pancakes are all made out of soft wheat flours.

Rice Flour

쌀가루 [ssalgaru]

When making rice cakes, rice noodles, and even kimchi, you will need rice flour. It is rich in calcium for bone health, and it has a high mineral density for an immunity boost. As with any flour, it is the quality of the rice grains to be milled that matters the most, so use organic rice flour if possible.

Rice flour is gluten-free, so it is a great choice for people who have autoimmune conditions such as celiac disease. It contains a healthy amount of insoluble fiber, which improves cardiovascular health and balances the digestive tract and blood sugar levels.

Rice powder is an essential ingredient for making kimchi. We mix rice powder with water, scoops of Korean hot pepper paste, and garlic to create a sticky paste for kimchi.

In addition to cooking with rice flour, it can be used as a natural skin exfoliant, removing dead skin and debris. Many Korean face masks include rice flour, which gets rid of dark circles and tightens the skin.

Multigrain Flour

Grandma would always come back from Korea with a black bag full of misugaru (미숫가루) powder, a traditional Korean multigrain powder made of brown rice, sweet rice, black soybeans, barley, perilla seeds, black sesame seeds, Job's tears, and quinoa. A scoop of powdered misugaru mixed with water and honey is the ultimate vegan protein shake before protein shakes existed. This mildly sweet and malty drink is truly a superfood that will keep you full and energized.

Misugaru, also called seonsik (선식), has been around for over a thousand years in Korea. This nutrient-dense mixture was used as a meal substitute back when food was scarce. Buddhist monks also drank a liquid form before they went into meditation to help their minds stay clear and calm. Today, people drink misugaru to try to consume a healthy amount of grains and fewer carbohydrates. It is now considered a diet meal replacement.

Mung Bean Starch

녹두 전분 [nokdu jeonbun]

Mung beans are an essential staple in Korean porridges and pancakes. They are also one of the best plant-based sources of protein. Mung bean starch is rich in amino acids and nutrient-dense antioxidants such as phenolic acids, flavonoids, and cinnamic acid that aid in digestive health and promote weight loss. Rich in potassium, magnesium, and fiber, these powerful beans can even lower blood pressure and blood sugar levels.

Perilla Seed Powder

들깨가루 [deulkkae-garu]

Made from ground perilla seeds, perilla powder has a deep, nutty, earthy taste with a touch of mint flavor. It is used to thicken and season Korean stews and soup as well as enhance the flavor of herbal dishes. Perilla seeds contain a high amount of omega-3s and are used to treat health issues such as induced sweating, asthma, nausea, and muscle spasms. Adding perilla seed powder to your stews with chives will bring balance between flavors, emotions, and organs in constant motion. It has an aromatic flavor and is used as a spice. The dense nutty flavor brings a warmth feeling and a sense of home.

Other flours to add to your pantry include acorn flour, barley malt flour, buckwheat flour, and green tea powder.

Fruits and Nuts for Longevity

Growing up, Umma would tell us fruits are spirit food and nuts are brain food. We need both to nourish and fuel our mind and spirit to live a long and healthy life. Instead of cake and chocolate desserts, a traditional Korean dessert would be fruit such as Korean pear, persimmons, Korean melon, Kyoho or Muscat grapes, and tea.

Jujube

대추 [daechu]

Jujube is a sweet treat and has been cultivated for more than four thousand years for its incredible healing abilities. The Korean jujube is small and oval with light green skin that becomes red-brown and wrinkly as the fruit ripens. By September and October, the jujube fruit is in peak season and can be found at farmers' markets and Asian grocery stores.

In Eastern medicine, the fruit is used to improve sleep and aid in digestion. The jujube contains flavonoids and saponins, which trigger the release of neurotransmitters that help with falling asleep and also with staying asleep. For centuries, jujubes have been eaten or brewed in tea for a peaceful night of sleep. The sedative effects have similar results on the mind and body.

In addition to its properties as a sleep aid, the fruit has been used to help relieve constipation and indigestion. The jujube fruit triggers GABA (gamma-aminobutyric acid) and serotonin, two critical neurotransmitters for regulating mood and relaxation. Studies have shown that the jujube fruit may have a calming effect on the brain and also relieves anxiety.

This tiny fruit packs a big punch when it comes to fighting inflammation and oxidative stress. The jujube fruit also has been used in traditional medicine to help reduce inflammation. With less inflammation, the body can strengthen its immune system and fight off illness and chronic disease.

The fruit can be consumed in a variety of ways: fresh, dried, boiled, and also in tea. It is rich in essential vitamins, minerals, and antioxidants. In 100 grams (3½ ounces) of jujube, there is about 69 milligrams of vitamin C. The fruit helps fight free radicals, boosts immunity, and helps keep skin healthy. The jujube is also high in fiber, making it great for digestion. Adding jujube to a hot tea of Qi Alchemy herbal pearls creates a terrific tonic to manage stress and improve digestion.

Pine Nuts

잣 [jat]

There is a Korean saying that three years of consuming pine nut porridge would lead one to become an immortal spirit because of its miraculous and fortifying medicinal properties. Pine nuts are a delicacy and are sprinkled in many teas as a garnish and used in desserts and porridges. They have a tonic effect that helps with digestion. They are full of antioxidants and contain vitamins A, B, C, D, and E. Pine nuts support healthy cholesterol levels and decrease appetite through the release of cholecystokinin, an appetite-suppressing hormone. Eating a handful of pine nuts goes a long way and may turn you into an immortal spirit.

Oils

기름 [gileum]

Our ancestors consumed oils that were fresh-pressed oils. These were not refined oils, such as vegetable oils and margarine, which have contributed to a dramatic increase in heart disease and other chronic conditions. Refined oils are depleted of the vitamins and minerals that occur naturally in the plant. For our bodies to metabolize their calories, we deplete stored nutrients in our tissues and bones. These refined oils have stripped our mineral content and have created an imbalance in the tissue levels of our essential fatty acids.

Sesame Oil

참기름 [chan gileum]

During the Joseon dynasty in the 1300s, kings enjoyed sesame oil, and the plant was grown to pay tribute to the king. Grindstones were used to extract the oil from sesame seeds. Korean sesame oil has unique aromatic characteristics. The amber color and smell come from roasting the sesame seeds. Variables such as temperature, time, humidity, and the right level of pressure are considered when producing quality sesame oil. Sesame oil is used in many herbal dishes and has a rich, nutty flavor.

Korean Chile Oil

한국 고추 기름 [hanguk gochu gileum]

Korean red chile peppers symbolize the sun, and its spicy flavors are said to cast away bad forces. Chile oil is a key ingredient in many spicy Korean dishes such as spicy tofu stew. A few tablespoons (45 to 60 ml) create a deep savory-tasting spice.

Perilla Oil

들깨 [deulkkae]

The smell of perilla leaves brings back fond memories of Grandma harvesting perilla leaves. We would harvest buckets full of perilla leaves, spread them on the ground, and start counting to fifty. Once fifty leaves were stacked, we would roll the leaves like rolling a wad of cash with a rubber band. Caterpillars and ladybugs would squirm and move among the perilla leaves, confused about where they were going. I would pick them up delicately with wooden chopsticks and release them back to the garden because it wasn't fair for them to leave their natural habitat. We would roll bundles and bundles each with fifty leaves until we created a big amount to sell to our local market.

Grandma was so pleased with us when we were done rolling perilla bundles. It took time, patience, and a great deal of squatting.

Perilla seeds contain the highest amount of omega-3 of any plant, and a tablespoon (15 ml) of perilla oil has roughly the same amount of alpha-linolenic acid from omega-3 as a whole mackerel. Perilla oil is a versatile, complex oil that brings out an earthy and nutty taste. Summer greens, such as watercress or dandelion greens, are great with perilla oil.

Plum Extract

실 원액 [maesil wonaek]

Plum extract, also known as green plum extract, has been used in Korea since ancient times for its antibacterial properties and its support in digestion. It is frequently used as a sugar substitute in Korean cuisine, adding a sweetness and tartness to a dish. It is great for salad dressings, marinades, and dipping sauces.

If you can find green plums in the spring, you can make the extract yourself by mixing equal parts of the plum and sugar in an airtight glass jar. Let it sit in a dark space at room temperature for at least 3 months. Then, strain the fruit out from the liquid and allow the liquid to ferment in an airtight jar for a year. It will age and form into a deep sweet-flavored syrup.

The plum fruits can be reused to make Korean plum soju (liquor) or plum vinegar by placing the fruit into another container. For plum soju, add equal amounts of plum and soju. For plum rice vinegar, add equal amounts of plum and rice vinegar. The plum syrup can also be consumed iced by adding water and ice!

Menstruum

용매 [yongmae]

Fermented rice wine is one of the vehicles, or menstruums, for extracting constituents and plant nutrients. The standard ratio of herb to rice wine is 1 part the weight of dried herb to 5 parts the volume of menstruum.

Korean Rice Wine

막걸리 [makgolli]

Korea's oldest alcoholic drink, makgolli (막걸리), is a yeast-fermented rice wine and was considered farmer's liquor. Makgolli and soju uses three simple ingredients: rice, water, and nuruk—a dry cake composed of bacteria, wild yeasts, and koji mold spores. Fermenting cooked nuruk, sweet rice, and water, the nuruk breaks down starch in the rice into sugar, creating a sweet alcohol mixture called wonju (원주). Once this mixture is settled, a top clear liquid is separated into a cheonju (청주) alcohol, which the Korean aristocrats drank. Once distilled, soju is made and the remaining settled sediment is diluted with water and roughly strained to make makgolli.

Soju

소주 [soju]

Soju literally means "burned liquor" as it is traditionally made by distilling alcohol from fermented grains.

During the Goryeo era in the fourteenth century, Korean alchemists learned Levantine distilling techniques from Arab tribes and developed their own distilling technique using rice and other grains, creating soju.

The rice wine for distilled soju is usually fermented for about fifteen days, and the distillation process involves boiling the filtered, mature rice wine in a sot (cauldron) topped with a soju gori (a two-storied distilling appliance with a pipe).

Rather than using alcohol, vinegars are a great way to make nutritive-dense tonic herbs. See the vinegar list on page 34 for building your apothecary.

Salts and Spices

소금과 향신료 [sogeumgwa hyangshinlyo]

Salts and spices are essential building blocks for creating your Korean apothecary. These contain large quantities of trace minerals and bring out the natural flavors of a dish. One ounce (20 g) of dried spices contains higher mineral content than fruits or vegetables. Importantly, salt, which is an essential ingredient in making kimchi, is used for preserving foods.

Korean Chile Pepper

고추가루 [gochugalu]

In Korean culture, the shape of the Korean chile pepper represents the birth of a male infant. The sun-dried spiciness of peppers elevates the heat and color of our stews, soups, and fermented foods, and it is one of the most important spices to have in our apothecary. The quality of the chile pepper can add spice and flavor to any dish.

Sesame Seeds

참깨 [chamkkae]

There is a legend about Korean sesame seeds, and it goes like this: Once there was a girl who was worried about her looks and her aging skin, so a friend suggested a simple organic treatment that would keep her skin soft and smooth. She eagerly went home and soaked her body with water and sesame seeds. Hours later, the girl's mother entered the bathroom and saw that the sesame seeds were

SESAME SOY DRESSING

참깨 간장 드레싱 [chamkkae ganjang deulesing]

**MAKES 2 TABLESPOONS
(28 ML)**

1 tablespoon (15 ml) soy
 sauce
1 teaspoon rice vinegar
1 teaspoon plum vinegar
½ teaspoon mirin
1 teaspoon sesame seeds

The fermented taste and ingredients of soy sauce is an important base in Korean cuisine and is based on the principles of the five flavors. This recipe is an easy way to enhance the taste of your dishes or to use as a dipping sauce.

1. Add the soy sauce, rice vinegar, plum vinegar, mirin, and sesame seeds to a small bowl. Whisk or stir with a fork to combine.

—

Small as a sesame seed, we are stewards of the earth.

attached to her daughter's body. The seeds had rooted themselves into the girl's skin.

Sesame seeds are a common Korean garnish. These seeds are one of the oldest-known oilseed crops in the world and are rich in protein, vitamins, minerals, and antioxidants.

Korean Solar Sea Salt

천일염 [cheon-il-yeom]

The Korean West Sea, also called The Yellow Sea and Hwang Hai, is the only mudflat that produces sea salt among the five largest mudflats in the world. The perfect conditions for producing high-quality solar sea salt are shallow waters, a large tidal range, and clean fresh air along with abundant sunrays. Mudflat sea salt is the original Korean traditional sea salt that's sun-dried. It is commonly infused with herbs such as garlic, thyme, basil, or mugwort to enhance the flavors of our food without compromising our health.

Hand-harvested by farmers, this salt (called jayeom) is rare. A complex method that has been passed down through generations of Koreans since the eighteenth century, the process involves boiling salt water in stone salt kilns until a bright white heated salt is produced. The solar method of salt farming first entered Korea under Japanese colonization in the 1900s. During that time, the mudflats were seized, and the majority of the salt produced was exported.

Shiitake Mushroom

표고버섯 [pyogo beoseos]

Shiitake mushroom, also called Lentinus edodes, is slightly warm, moist, a stimulant, and a nutritive tonic because of its beta-glucans. The caps and stems are used, and it is an immune balancer. Dried shiitake mushrooms are easy to find at Asian markets and have a long shelf life. We all need a little shiitake in our herbal cuisines and broths.

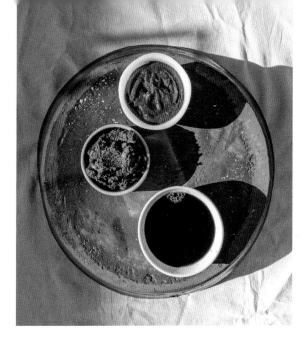

Fermented Pastes

발효 반주 [balhyo banjook]

Soybean fermentation is rich in flavonoids and beneficial vitamins, minerals, and phytoestrogens. Certain compounds in fermented soy, such as genistein, may help reduce the risk of certain cancers like breast and color cancer.

Fermented Soybean Paste

된장 [doenjang]

Meju bricks are the standard process of many fermented herbal foods in Korea, such as soy sauce, doenjang (fermented soybean paste), and gochujang (Korean red chile paste). The ritual of meju fermentation started in the Three Kingdoms around 50 BCE. The soybeans are thoroughly washed and then boiled, mashed, and molded into meju bricks. The meju bricks are then tied with rice straw and hung in a cool, shaded area to solidify and ferment. While they are air-drying, the rice stalks infuse *Bacillus subtilis* bacteria into the meju bricks.

Doenjang is made traditionally with only two natural ingredients: soybean and sea salt. This salt-of-the-earth paste goes through a slow fermentation process and doesn't need any added ingredients to produce a deep, rich, and savory flavor. The salt is dried and aged for at least three years before being used to remove the bitterness in the salt crystals and deepen the flavor.

The fermented bricks of soybeans are stored in an earthenware pot called onggi (옹기), where they will sit outside and slowly age for up to one thousand days. The result is a deeply savory and traditional-tasting doenjang.

Fermented Red Chile Paste

고추장 [gochujang]

To add more variety to a bowl of rice and aid in digestion, sun-dried red pepper was fermented and then bound with rice flour to make gochujang chile paste. It is left to ferment in a large onggi for twelve months and up to many years. The fermented red chile paste is abundant in nutrients including vitamins B_2 and C, protein, and carotenes. Gochujang, along with kimchi, is one of Korea's most recognized fermented foods.

Fermented Soybean and Red Chile Paste

쌈장 [ssamjang]

Ssamjang tastes like a blend of fermented soybean paste and red chile paste that's mildly spicy and salty, with a slight hint of garlic. It is the perfect dipping paste for fresh veggies, lettuce or perilla wraps, and grilled meat.

Sauces

소스 [soseu]

There's a Korean proverb, "Food is only as good as the jang." Korean sauces, or jang, are rich in depth and complexity. From sweet to nutty and savory, its natural fermentation process is the secret behind the diverse flavors.

Soy Sauce

간장 [ganjang]

There is a saying that "the happiness of the family depends on the taste of soy sauce" because of the patient and long fermentation process of brewing soy sauce and its various phases. Soybeans, water, wheat, and salt are mixed together to ferment. The bitter molecules found in salt crystals separate and float to the top and are then skimmed off, reducing the saltiness and the slightly bitter aftertaste. The soybeans are mashed into meju bricks and left to ferment for six months. After the soy sauce is extracted, it is left to age for another full year to develop a rich, full-bodied flavor.

Soy products are among the most popular foods in Asia, and there have been studies that soy consumption contributes to positive health and longevity of the Korean and Japanese population. Soy is rich in both minerals and essential fatty acids and contains hormone-like substances that can reduce menopausal symptoms.

Fish Sauce

생선 소스 [saengseon soseu]

We always need a spoonful of umami whenever a stew tastes like something is missing. Umami flavor in Korean is called gamchil-mat (감칠맛). Fish sauce is usually boiled with other Korean ingredients such as dashima (seaweed), shiitake mushrooms, onions, and Korean radish to produce a rich-flavored fish sauce.

TOOLS

We are pressed on every side by the troubles of this world, but as herbalists, we are not scattered. We are perplexed but not driven to despair. Tools are our vessels to preserve and store our bespoke herbal apothecary.

Moon Jars

달항아리 [dalhangari]

Moon jars are made out of milky-white porcelain and resemble the full moon. A skilled potter combines the top and bottom halves of the moon and places it in a fiery kiln through the fire that bakes it at about 1,832°F (1,000°C).

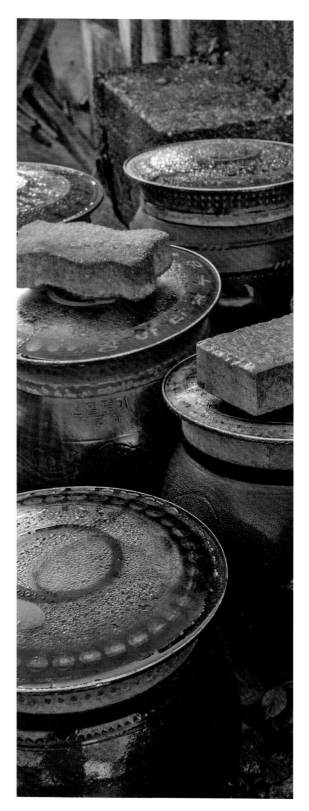

As the upper and lower halves are joined together, they come alive as one unit, becoming a full moon. Inside the jar holds the vitality Qi that enables new sprouts of spring to push their way through frozen winter ground. Originally created during the Joseon dynasty in the 1300s, they are curvaceous, pure white porcelain jars that customarily were made to contain flowers or wine. They are also ritual, votive vessels. The moon jar is simply pure.

Earthenware Jars

토기 항아리 [togi hangari]

Earthenware jars, hangari (항아리) or onggi (옹기), are fermenting vessels. Hangari are used for flowers or wine, and they are also used for ritual, votive vessels. Onggi earthenware is used as tableware and storage containers in Korea. They are usually located outside on a terrace near the kitchen and are used to store or ferment food such as kimchi, soybeans, grains, and bean and red pepper paste. Key conditions such as sunshine and air circulation play a large part in where the earthenware jar is placed so that the contained food is preserved and kept fresh. Sometimes, well-preserved ingredients like soy sauce may be contained in the earthenware jar for several years.

Kamasot Iron Pot

쇠 가마솥 [sae-kamasoteu]

Kamasot was the main iron pot used when making soups and rice, and it was considered the most important piece of cookware during the Three Kingdom era. *Kama* means "furnace" and *sot* means "pot." The kama takes considerable time to heat because of its low level of thermal conductivity. It absorbs and retains heat very well, thoroughly cooking the ingredients in the pot. When moving to a new house, the first piece to place in the kitchen was the kama. This ritual symbolized the establishment of a sharing home by families who share meals from the same kama.

Other Tools for Your Apothecary

- Small and large mason jars or amber glass jars
- Mortar and pestle
- Empty heat-and-seal tea bags
- Muslin bags
- Digital kitchen scale
- 1-ounce (28 ml) and 2-ounce (60 ml) dropper bottles for travel-sized tinctures
- Straw baskets for collecting and drying herbs
- Wooden and metal spoon and chopsticks

DRIED HERBS

말린 약초 [mallin yakcho]

Your herbal apothecary should include mugwort, seaweed, garlic, chives, ginger, and turmeric or curcumin. We will take a closer look at these herbs in the next chapter.

CORNERSTONE OF OUR HEARTS

Disease is in essence the result of conflict between soul and mind, so understanding the nature of disease is critical. We each have a soul, which is our real self, and our soul knows what experiences and knowledge can be obtained from our environment. Let herbs access every corner of your heart so that when we create herbal formulas for ourselves or others, flavor, function, feeling, love, and beauty should all be considered.

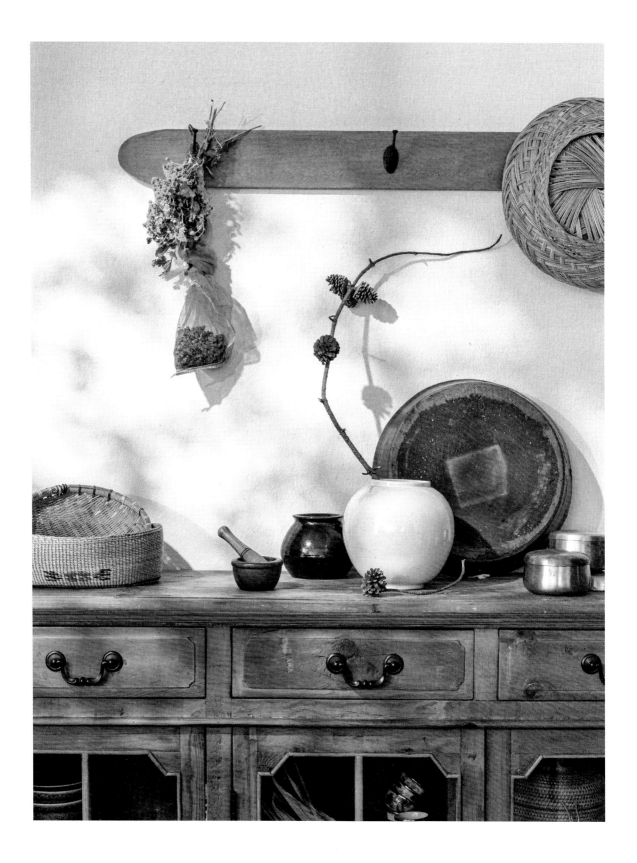

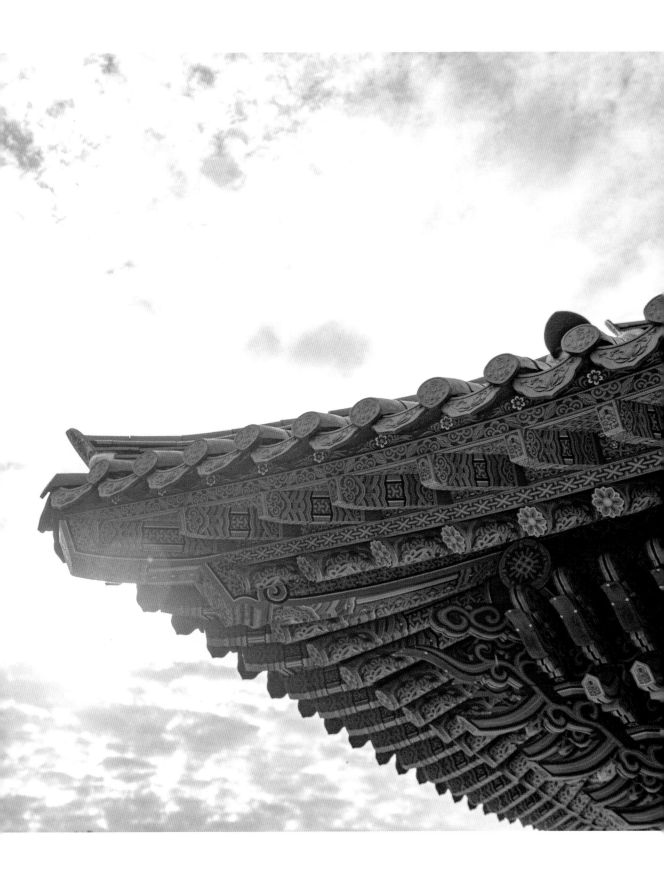

4 HEAVEN HERBS OF SPRING

☰ 건 [geon]

Man-root
A farmer's son playing his sweet harmonica to family ginseng roots
Bean sprouts like musical notes creating melodies and trailing in the air
His father hears the tunes of his son's harmonica and runs
Birds stop chirping and bean sprouts fall to the ground
Teardrops trickle down the rice paddy as his father threw the harmonica away
Know your roots and be a man, father said
Head down, the farmer's son went back to his ginseng bed nestled under a mound of hay
Sleep and dream a little longer, so his roots become a man

My father was a farmer's son in Paju, South Korea, and I always yearned to understand his childhood. He had to leave his family at nine years old to go to school in Seoul. Whenever I'm at our farm within the ancestral homelands of Paju, I pass by my family burial mounds, and I see the architecture of relationships and the shimmering threads of spiderwebs that hold it all together. Ancestral stories need to be unearthed as a reminder of respect to our native land.

HEAVEN FOLKTALE: PEOPLE OF MUGWORT AND GARLIC

When we think of our land and how much it has evolved throughout the years, we pay homage to the Dangun (단군) for giving us our native land. Long ago, the God of the Heavens, Hwanin (환인), had a son, Hwanung (환웅), who had a strong desire to rule the earth. As he gazed down at the mountains of the earth from the Heavens, Hwanung asked his father if he could descend upon the earth and rule over it. His father granted his son's wish and sent him down with a group of three thousand beings and brought the gods of rain, wind, and clouds with him to Earth. They descended to Shindansu, the Holy Tree of Life, on Mount Taebaek, where he began overseeing human world affairs such as food, life, disease, punishment, and morality.

After Hwanung continued to lead the earth, a bear and a tiger prayed to Hwanung and expressed their desire to become humans. Upon hearing their wishes, Hwanung gave them herbs—mugwort (*Artemisia vulgaris*) and garlic (*Allium sativum*)—and told the bear and the tiger, "If you avoid sunlight for 100 days and only eat garlic and mugwort, I will grant your wish." After agreeing, the bear and the tiger took up residence in a cave.

Many days passed. The tiger was feeling deprived and fled the cave, while the bear persevered and survived in the cave for 100 days. Hwanung kept his promise and transformed the bear into a woman, who was named Ungnyeo (웅녀), Bear Woman.

Ungnyeo became lonely and sad that she did not have a companion, so she prayed again to Hwanung for a son. Moved by her prayers, Hwanung transformed himself into a human and married Ungnyeo. They had a son and named him Dangun.

As the first human prince of the land, Dangun eventually established his own kingdom. This kingdom was called Gojoseon (고조선) (Ancient Joseon) and became the first Korean kingdom. The Dangun folktale represents the union

of nature—the God of Heaven and Mother Earth—and the importance of nature and the cosmos.

Koreans have traditionally used herbs since ancient times for health and dietary reasons and also for rituals in restoring balance and casting out evil spirits. In the folktale, mugwort and garlic are essential herbs that Koreans use and have many health benefits, such as improving immunity and sleep, as well as reducing inflammation and supporting blood flow.

Mugwort 쑥 [ssuk]

FAMILY: Asteraceae

GENUS: *Artemisia vulgaris*

COMMON NAMES: mugwort, felon herb, wild wormwood

PARTS USED: herb, roots

EFFECTIVE QUALITIES: pungent, bitter, aromatic, dry, cool, stimulating, restoring

NATIVE REGIONS: Eastern Asia, Europe

CONSTITUENTS: flavonoids, essential oil, coumarin derivatives, resin, tannins

PROPERTIES: complex temperature with cooling bitter principles and warming aromatics, drying, strong vital stimulant, astringent, aromatic, bitter tonic, mild choleretic, antimicrobial, antispasmodic

INDICATED USES: digestive issues, menstruation, parasites

NUTRIENTS: polyunsaturated fatty acids, phenolic compounds, vitamin C, essential amino acids

—

PREPARATION: Mugwort is prepared by infusion, tincture, or culinary form. Externally, it is used as washes, sitz baths, or suppositories.

DOSE: Infusion: 3–8 grams; tincture: 1–3 milliliters at 1:3 strength in 45 percent ethanol

CAUTION: Due to its emmenagogue action, mugwort should not be used during pregnancy. It may also cause an allergic reaction in individuals with existing allergies.

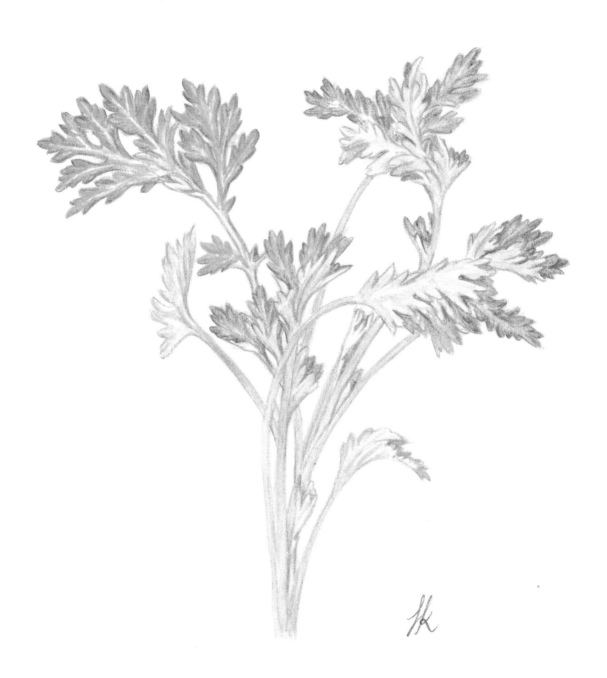

—

In America, mugwort is considered to be a weed, but in Korea, mugwort has a long history of Korean lore and has been used in folk herbal medicine, especially for the womb. It is commonly used for calming nerves, soothing menstrual pains, and promoting sleep, and it is a spiritual herb. With more than seventy-five unique chemicals, it is used to purify spaces in a similar way to incense and has a well-known effect on dreams. Mugwort is versatile and used to add flavor to herbal vinegars, seasonings, and tea. Externally, mugwort is used for body care (e.g., bath soaks) and incense.

In Eastern medicine, mugwort is used in a practice called moxibustion, which uses dried mugwort on particular points of the body to stimulate Qi, the flow of energy. Mugwort is usually placed on the skin with an acupuncture needle attached. The herb is then triggered and released with heat as it discharges toxins from the body. The healing properties of mugwort in this manner help release toxins from our body, and we can feel the benefits almost immediately by feeling our muscles relax or having quality sleep.

Mugwort is considered a dream herb and often is used to address sleep issues. It has a sweet and floral scent, making it excellent for use in aromatherapy. Its aromatic qualities are used during ceremonies and meditation practices. Keep in mind that mugwort is not going to solve all your sleep problems or have your lucid dreams come true. Having a nighttime ritual before bed, such as meditating, visualizing, or breathwork, can make a difference in enhancing your dreams and tracking your sleep progress.

When mugwort is consumed, it supports digestion and has relaxing properties that decongest the liver, improve appetite, and calm the stomach. It also harmonizes your monthly moon cycle and decongests stomach Qi stagnation. The combination of mugwort's antiseptic and anti-inflammatory actions treat intestinal and urinary tract infections.

Inner Beauty Reflection

To create a peaceful society through behaviors and attitudes, Koreans set intentions on our daily habits—everything from our skin-care routine, bath culture, eating habits, and spiritual practice. Clean and soft skin is considered beautiful in Confucianism as it shows that prudence and modesty develop internal beauty rather than external beauty. Instead of a painted makeup face, the focus was on natural beauty—having a clear and healthy face.

Bathhouses in Korea called jimjilbang (찜질방) are an essential part of our culture for holistic health and keeping our skin clean. From hot- and cold-temperature stone caves to wet and dry rooms, the spaces are heated with charcoal and the walls are installed with various natural elements such as woods, minerals, stones, salts, and metals. There are multiple bathtubs that are soaked with herbal ingredients such as mugwort or calendula. Korean kiln saunas were used for traditional medicinal purposes and were maintained by Buddhist monks.

Beauty from the inside out is a reflection of how we take care of our skin health and lifestyle. Skin, our largest organ, plays an important role for our overall health. It warms our body and holds our body fluids, protects us from harmful microbes, and allows us to feel. The feelings of warmth, cold, and sometimes pain come from our skin sensation. We must be mindful of the ways we protect, exfoliate, and apply certain ingredients on our body, which will have lasting effects on the earth. Being aware of the ingredients that are used in products makes us conscious consumers and helps us lean toward the Confucian philosophy on beauty: Less is more. We live in a world where overconsumption is ruining our environment and has reduced our ecosystem. Can we reduce the amount of skin-care products we use? What lifestyle practices have improved my skin? Going back to the basics like quality sleep, hydration, exfoliating, and a healthy balanced diet are true solutions to improving skin. My 65-year-old aunt in Korea has the smoothest glowing skin, and her skin-care secret is happiness and a big brimmed hat. This routine has worked for my aunt, but each of us has our own way of protecting and enhancing our skin care. There is no one set solution.

MUGWORT TEA

쑥차 [ssukcha]

Makes 1 cup (235 ml) of tea

1 to 1½ teaspoons dried mugwort
1 cup (235 ml) water

Brew this simple mugwort tea before bed and take deep breaths before drinking the tea. As we end our night, we sip on mugwort tea to dispel any wind or pain. We close our eyes and give gratitude for the day, and we ask the Heavens to give us sweet dreams. Let mugwort guide us to release any tension or pain and to liberate us from any fear or anxiety that keeps us up at night. It also helps us to have visionary peaceful dreams.

1. Place the mugwort in a teapot. Boil the water over high heat and then remove from the heat and pour the water over the mugwort.

2. Infuse the mugwort for about 8 to 10 minutes and then strain. Enjoy this herbaceous, detoxing drink.

—

Forgetting what is behind and straining toward what is ahead, we are joyful in the moment.

ॐ

NOTE: For the mugwort in this recipe, use fresh mugwort leaves dried overnight or purchase dried mugwort. For daily use, this tea can be enjoyed up to five times per day.

MUGWORT GREENS

쑥나물 [ssuk namul]

Serves 4

10 ounces (280 g) freshly harvested mugwort, trimmed and washed
1 tablespoon (8 g) sesame seeds, plus more for garnish
½ tablespoon sea salt
1½ tablespoons (25 ml) soy sauce
2 tablespoons (28 ml) sesame oil
1 teaspoon minced garlic
Cooked multigrain rice, for serving

This simple and nourishing herbal dish combines essential Korean culinary ingredients that are useful for everyday cooking.

1. Bring water to a boil in a medium saucepan over medium-high heat. Blanch the mugwort in the boiling water for 5 to 7 minutes. Strain through a fine-mesh sieve and squeeze out the water from the mugwort.

2. In a small bowl, combine the sesame seeds, salt, soy sauce, sesame oil, and garlic and then add the mugwort. Gently massage all the ingredients.

3. Garnish the greens with sesame seeds for an extra dose of sesame flavor. Serve on a bed of multigrain rice.

—

I breathe in and out, feeling myself breathing but not trying to control or regulate my breath. I let go, and the harmony of my breath feels effortless.

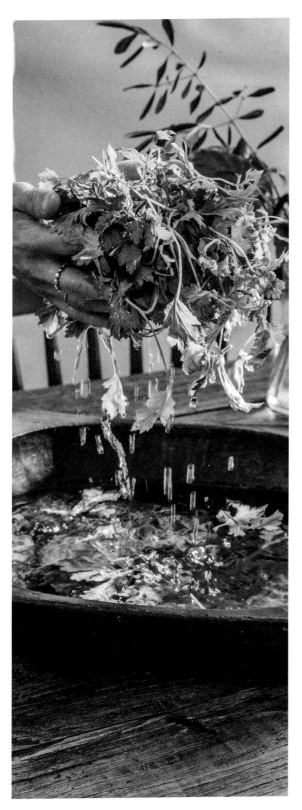

Essential nutrients and antioxidants like glutathione, carotenoids, and vitamins A, E, and C help protect the skin against sun damage and anti-aging effects. Our skin cells need to receive enough nutrients to regenerate new cells. By fighting free radicals, vitamins A and C can help stop the breakdown of collagen, the protein responsible for skin structure and repair. Unfortunately, the foods we eat may not allow us to receive adequate nutrients, so supplements may be helpful when we are deficient. Most Americans are deficient in vitamins D, E, and A and magnesium and calcium, so it's important to get nutrient panel blood tests on a regular basis.

As we age, our bodies slowly stop producing collagen, so taking vitamins A and C slow the breakdown of collagen and can help repair damaged skin from free radicals caused by pollution and sunlight. Herbs such as jujube (page 52), wolfberry (goji berry, page 34), and ginseng (page 71) are rich in nutrients and help improve skin health.

Acne is one of the most common skin issues and is derived from hormonal imbalance and stress. Herbs that regulate the adrenal glands like red ginseng, ashwagandha, rhodiola, or holy basil can help reduce stress levels, causing less acne breakouts. Herbs such as maca root, willow bark, and dandelion can help balance hormones and treat pimples.

Ultimately, whatever is seen externally is a reflection of your internal health, and a large part of skin health has to do with a healthy liver. Not only is acne a result of hormonal imbalance and stress, it can also represent a damaged and unhealthy gut or liver; therefore, taking herbal teas and staying hydrated with water is a great place to begin. Our liver is a critical organ that works endlessly to support our immunity and metabolism, cleaning toxins out of our blood. Bitter herbs such as mugwort (page 62) generate the liver's metabolic process, reducing acne. Other herbs like burdock root, yellow dock, milk thistle, and dandelion root have stimulating and decongesting properties that protect the liver. Eliminating refined sugars, soda, and processed foods can also drastically improve your skin health.

MUGWORT YONI STEAM OR BATH SOAK

쑥 목욕 [ssuk mokyok]

MAKES 1 STEAM OR SOAK

3 cups (700 ml) water
⅔ cup (32 g) fresh or dried mugwort

Mugwort baths are one of the best ways to soothe your skin, relax your muscles, and elevate your mood. A self-care ritual that Koreans use to cleanse their uterus and balance the monthly moon cycle is yoni steaming with mugwort. One of my favorite ways to enjoy mugwort is creating an herbal bath. When taking a bath, having rituals like lighting candles around the tub and playing soft music creates a meditative vibe.

1. Bring the water to a boil. Fill a 24-ounce (680 ml) mason jar with the fresh and dried mugwort. Add the boiling water to the herbs, cover, and steep the herbs for at least 20 minutes.

2. For a yoni steam, pour the herbs and hot water in a pot and sit over the pot and wrap a towel over your waist for the steam to enter your vulva for about 20 minutes. Be careful to keep a safe distance between the pot and your skin.

3. For a bath, once the mugwort has been steeped, strain through a fine-mesh sieve and pour the mugwort infusion into your bath. Soak in your own intuition and enjoy the flow of a cleansing bath.

—

I will let go of the toxic ties that are preventing me from growing and thriving.

Garlic 마늘 [maneul]

FAMILY: Amaryllidaceae

GENUS: *Allium sativum*

COMMON NAMES: garlic bulb, poor man's treacle

PART USED: root

EFFECTIVE QUALITIES: pungent, aromatic, hot, very dry, somewhat salty, stimulating, dispersing, decongesting, diluting, strong diffusive, mild relaxant

NATIVE REGION: worldwide

CONSTITUENTS: trace elements, enzymes, sulfurous compounds, essential oils, phytohormones

PROPERTIES: antiseptic, heating immune-enhancing alternative, stimulating expectorant, diaphoretic

INDICATED USES: antiseptic, warms the lungs, promotes expectoration, resolves phlegm, warms the stomach, promotes digestion, relieves bloating

NUTRIENTS: vitamins A, B, and C

—

PREPARATION: Garlic is used in culinary dishes or taken in tincture or other extract form. Tincture from fresh or freshly dried clove helps treat numerous internal and external conditions.

DOSE: Raw clove: 3 cloves. Up to 8 cloves a day may be taken in acute conditions like an infection. Tincture: 0.5–2 milliliters at 1:3 strength in 45 percent ethanol.

CAUTION: Due to its hot, dry qualities, garlic is very stimulating. It should not be used during pregnancy and breastfeeding. Garlic may also cause flatulence in sensitive stomachs.

—

Pungent and heating, garlic is a universal herb and a nutrient powerhouse used to cleanse the blood, among other things. It is a stimulant, antimicrobial, and expectorant, making it great for colds and moving mucus out of the body.

Stimulation is promoted in congestive cold syndromes, such as heart yang deficiency. By warming the interior and dispelling cold, garlic eliminates chronic damp conditions. Garlic warms the stomach and lungs, promotes digestion, decongests the liver, promotes bile flow, balances blood sugar levels, and stimulates the immune system. Garlic may be small, but it is full of vitamins B and C, iron, copper, potassium, manganese, and selenium.

With significant antibacterial properties, garlic helps protect against certain infections and also promotes heart health. This leads to overall protection for the heart by reducing cholesterol and lowering blood pressure. In fact, it has been found that those who have lower blood pressure are more likely to have consumed garlic in their diet.

recipe follows

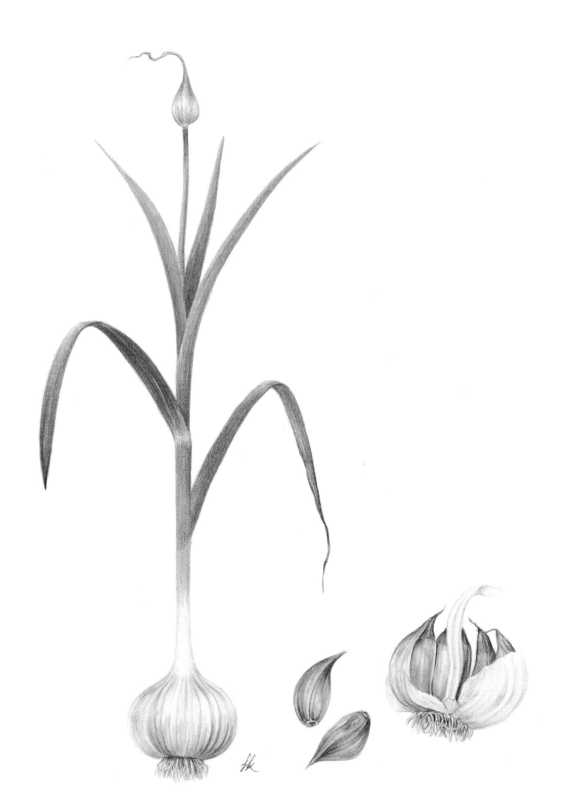

FERMENTED GARLIC CLOVES

발효 마늘 [balhyo maneul]

MAKES 1 PINT (473 ML)

5 garlic bulbs
1 cup (235 ml) water
2 tablespoons (28 ml) white or brown rice vinegar
2 tablespoons (28 ml) soy sauce
2 tablespoons (40 g) honey
2 tablespoons (28 ml) cooking wine
Pinch of salt

Koreans use garlic in almost all of their cuisine. This delicious, healthy side dish can be stored in the refrigerator for months. It is great to eat year-round and will keep your immune system healthy.

1. Peel the garlic cloves and transfer them to a clean glass 16-ounce (475 ml) mason jar.

2. Heat the water, vinegar, soy sauce, honey, and cooking wine in a small pot over medium heat. Bring to a boil and then let the mixture cool. Add a pinch of salt. Once the mixture is at room temperature, pour the mixture into the mason jar with the garlic and cover with a lid.

3. Let it sit in a dark room or pantry for at least 1 week to ferment and then transfer the mason jar to the fridge.

—

Protect me from the stresses of life and repair any oxidative damage.

NOTE: As with all herbs and gifts from Mother Earth, consume in moderation and show gratitude by eating or drinking with mindfulness. Overconsuming anything may develop dependence and can lead to addiction. If you are feeling any nausea, vomiting, dizziness, irritation, or inflammation in the mouth, throat, or skin, please seek medical attention.

Panax Ginseng 인삼 [insam]

FAMILY: Araliaceae

GENUS: *Panax ginseng*

COMMON NAMES: Korean ginseng, red ginseng, Asian ginseng, human root, life root

PART USED: root

EFFECTIVE QUALITIES: sweet, somewhat bitter, warm, slightly moist, tonic, Yang herb

NATIVE REGION: Central Asia

CONSTITUENTS: triterpenoid saponins, flavonoids, panaxadiol, sterols, essential oil, polyamines, nitrogenous compounds, enzymes, polysaccharides

PROPERTIES: adaptogenic, increases plasma levels of corticosterone (hormone involved in stress response), nootropic, liver protective, antioxidant, anti-inflammatory

INDICATED USES: relieves headaches, protects liver, alters hormone levels, promotes digestion, builds immunity, improves lungs, regulates blood sugar. Internally, it is used as an invigorator for fatigue, stress, depression, and decreased cognitive function. It exerts beneficial effects on the cardiovascular system and respiratory tract.

NUTRIENTS: vitamins A, E, and B_{12}, calcium, manganese, potassium, magnesium

—

PREPARATION: Red ginseng root is prepared by steaming the whole root or sliced root. It is taken in decoction, tincture, or elixir form.

DOSE: Decoction: 1–8 grams. The average dose is 2 grams. Tincture: 0.25–3 milliliters at 1:3 strength in 55 percent ethanol. The average dose is 1 milliliter.

CAUTION: Panax ginseng should not be used during pregnancy or breastfeeding. Individuals with high blood pressure, heart conditions, or autoimmune disease should not take ginseng.

—

Ginseng, considered the King of All Herbs or the Herb of Longevity, is a sacred herb native to Korea since 2000 BCE. Korea is known to harvest the best ginseng in the world due to its moist, shade-loving forest and mountainous terrain. It is a perennial herb that's 2 (61 cm) or more feet high with dark green leaves and red clusters of berries.

The valuable medical properties are in the root of the plant. It has unique compounds called ginsenosides, a class of saponins that are phytochemicals found in certain herbs containing powerful antibacterial properties. They boost our immune system, improve cardiovascular health, and reduce the risk of cancer. The medicinal effects and quality in ginseng are based not on its size but its shape. Ginseng roots that resemble a balanced human-shaped body with a head, body, arms, and legs are considered the best quality.

Korean red ginseng is cultivated for at least five years before being harvested. It goes through a hot-cold steaming and fermentation process to maximize the amount of saponins concentrated in each root. A healthy ginseng root has two to three thick main roots, a perfect "human body" shape, no red or black spots, and has many fine roots still intact.

With powerful healing properties, ginseng is world-renowned for its ability to tonify Qi, support the immune system, boost brain function, relieve fatigue and stress, increase energy and virility, as well as lower inflammation. Many of my clients who have chronic health conditions feel the benefits of red ginseng, but the herb should be considered both a preventive and remedial agent. Koreans treasure this sacred herb and consume ginseng on a regular basis as it is known to support overall health, vitality, and longevity.

recipes follow

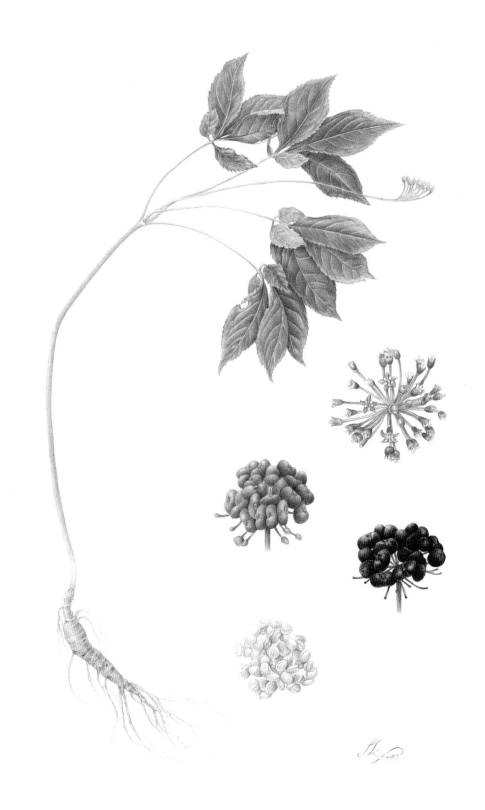

GINSENG HERBAL HONEY

인삼 꿀 [insam kkul]

MAKES 2 CUPS (680 G)

3 to 4 raw ginseng roots
2 cups (680 g) organic
  honey

Herbal-infused honey is one of my favorite ways to take herbs because the use of honey is common in sweetening many of our foods and it has a long shelf life. Whenever you need a boost of energy or need to relieve stress or fatigue, add ginseng herbal honey to your dish or tea.

1. Cut the raw ginseng into thin slices. Fill at least one-third of a 32-ounce (946 ml) mason jar with raw ginseng slices. Pour in enough organic honey to cover the ginseng slices. Place the mason jar of ginseng and honey in a dark pantry to ferment for at least 48 hours.

2. When it is ready, add a tablespoon (20 g) of the ginseng honey to 1½ cups (355 ml) of hot water to make ginseng herbal honey tea.

—

Protect my liver and energize my Qi, as I add ginseng honey to my tea.

GINSENG JUJUBE TEA

인삼 대추 차 [insam daechu cha]

MAKES 6 CUPS (1.4 L) OF TEA

2 raw ginseng roots
  (about the size of an
  index card)
10 dried jujubes
12 cups (2.8 L) water
Glass or clay pot

If you are feeling tired or stressed, use this tea to nourish the liver and blood and to tonify digestive and lung Qi.

1. Thoroughly wash and strain the ginseng and jujubes. Add the ginseng, jujubes, and water to a medium pot. Bring it to a boil for decoction. Reduce the heat and let it simmer until the volume of water is reduced by half. Strain through a fine-mesh strainer and transfer liquid to a 64-ounce (1.9 L) mason jar.

2. The tea can be served hot or cold. Add ginseng herbal honey (above) for an extra dose of ginseng sweetness.

—

Empty out the old to bring in a full and overflowing taste to enter.

NOTE: I usually mix the herbs in ½ to 1 cup (120 to 235 ml) of vinegar and water and then allow them to soak for about 20 minutes. Herbs for teas should be free of impurities to ensure the best taste. Drain the water and give the herbs a quick rinse.

Korean Pasque Flower
할미꽃 [halmi-kott]

FAMILY: Ranunculaceae

GENUS: *Pulsatilla koreana Nakai*

COMMON NAME: grandmother flower

PART USED: root

EFFECTIVE QUALITIES: cool, strong vital stimulant, relaxant

NATIVE REGION: native to Korea in open wastelands and grassy fields

CONSTITUENTS: saponins and anemonin. Saponins have been shown to decrease blood lipids, lower cancer risks, and lower blood glucose response. Anemonin has both cardiotoxic and cardiotonic properties.

PROPERTIES: anti-inflammatory, contraceptive, antiparasitic, antibacterial, antiamoebic, sedative

INDICATED USES: vaginal health, treats dysentery and scrofula

—

CAUTION: Please consult your Eastern medicine practitioner or healthcare provider before using pasque flowers as it may have contraindications. Fresh pasque flowers are very toxic and should never be ingested. Prolonged contact can cause skin irritations. Pasque flower should not be used during pregnancy.

—

A hairy, wispy perennial herb, the Korean pasque flower is a treasured native herb. It is called the grandmother flower. Its leaves are white and long-stalked and in a rose shape. The fruit heads have long feather styles.

There was once a widow who had two daughters. The older daughter married a wealthy man, but the younger daughter married a man who just made enough money to make ends meet. Once a woman is married into a new family, she is no longer part of her immediate family. As the widow got older, she went to visit each daughter. When she arrived at the older daughter's home, she was not welcomed and so she went on to see her younger daughter. As the widow traveled over many mountains almost close enough to see her daughter, she collapsed from fatigue and exhaustion and died. Several hours later, the young daughter found her deceased mother and, devastated, buried her body near her house. As spring came the following year, a unique flower bloomed on her grave. The flower had white tufts of hair and a hunched back resembling her old mother. Since then, the Korean pasque flower symbolizes the reincarnation of the dead widow, calling it granny flower.

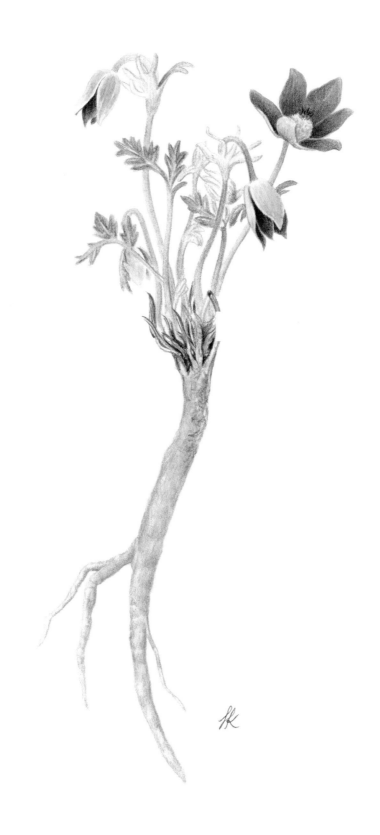

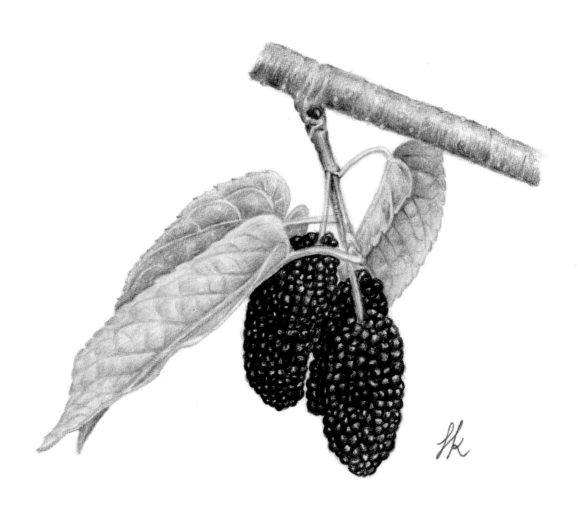

Mulberry 뽕나무 [ppongnamoo]

FAMILY: Moraceae

GENUS: *Morus alba*

COMMON NAME: white mulberry

PARTS USED: leaf, bark, fruit, root

EFFECTIVE QUALITIES: mild antihyperglycemic effect

NATIVE REGIONS: Korea, Central China, East China

CONSTITUENTS: organic acids (malic and citric acids), flavonoids, minerals, pectin

PROPERTIES: mild laxative, acidulous, antimicrobial

INDICATED USES: The leaf is used for hypertension and weakness. The bark is used for cough, dysuria, and constipation.

NUTRIENTS: vitamin C

PREPARATION: Mulberry is taken in a decoction or powder form. The leaves are usually used as tea.

—

DOSE: 4–10 grams of mulberry leaves

CAUTION: There are no reports of contraindications or side effects when used properly, but it should be noted that it has the possibility to lower blood sugar levels and is high in potassium.

—

Have you seen a tree with a milky sap? Most likely it is a member of the Mulberry family. A deciduous tree with smooth branches, the mulberry tree grows in the mountainous woods of Korea. Its leaves were feedstock for silkworms as well as making tea and folk remedies. Korean mulberry leaf tea is fairly sweet and is a great alternative to green tea. Rich in flavonoids, amino acids, and vitamin B complex, mulberry has medicinal healing properties. Internally, it is used as a mulberry syrup for feverish states and minor constipation. Externally, it is used as a mouthwash for throat or mouth inflammations.

PPONG MOUTHWASH

뽕 구강 청결제 [ppong gugang cheong-gyeolje]

MAKES 10 TO 12 USES

1 cup (6 to 10 g) organic mulberry leaf
1 cup (235 ml) hot water
1 ounce (28 ml) organic chrysanthemum extract
½ ounce (15 ml) organic calendula extract
¼ ounce (7 ml) white oak bark extract
¼ ounce (7 ml) myrrh extract

Oral care keeps bacteria from growing into infections and gum disease. We treasure the mulberry leaf with its many antibacterial efficacies, such as reducing inflammation, clearing heat, and stopping bleeding and pain.

1. Add the mulberry leaf to the hot water and steep for 20 minutes. Cool the tea to room temperature. Combine all the liquids and bottle it in an amber bottle for UV light protection. Refrigerate the bottle for 10 to 14 days before use.

—

We wait for our everbearing mulberry trees with calculated patience and care.

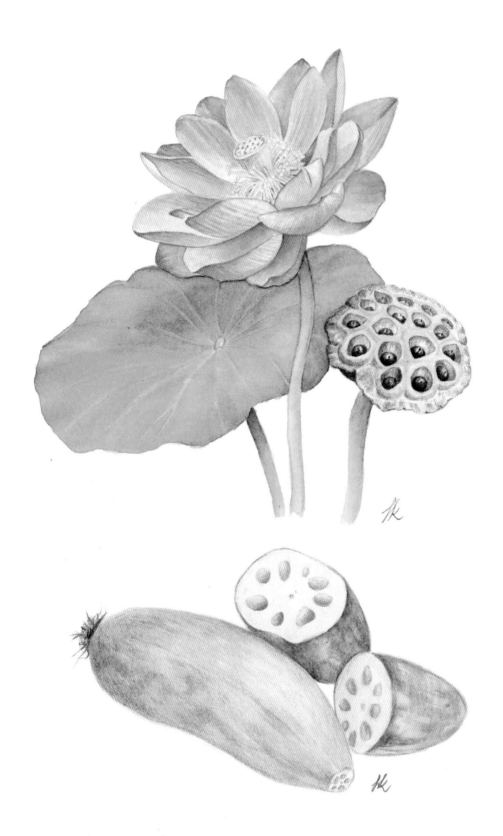

Sacred Lotus 연꽃 [yeonkkot]

FAMILY: Nelumbonaceae

GENUS: *Nelumbo nucifera*

COMMON NAMES: lotus, water lily

PARTS USED: rhizomes, seed

EFFECTIVE QUALITIES: astringent, relaxant, tonic

NATIVE REGIONS: South Asia, Middle East

CONSTITUENTS: sesquiterpenoids, essential oils, alkaloids, flavonoids

PROPERTIES: antidiabetic, anti-inflammatory, hypotensive

INDICATED USES: vasodilation, uterine, muscle relaxation, relieves hypertension

NUTRIENTS: trace elements of calcium, magnesium, iron, and zinc

—

PREPARATION: Lotus stems are often prepared in culinary dishes like salads. Dried lotus flowers are used in cooked dishes, and fresh lotus flowers are beautiful for decoration. Lotus seeds are usually in powdered form.

DOSE: For lotus seeds, use 3–10 grams of crushed or powdered seed, boiled in water for use as a decoction. Decoction for lotus stamen is 1.5–6 grams.

CAUTION: Those who are constipated or bloated should not ingest lotus as well as anyone with diabetes as it can lower blood sugar levels. The root should not be eaten raw since there is a risk of parasitic infection.

—

Grown widely throughout Asia, this large aquatic herb has thick rhizomes rooted in muddy water, yet it blossoms beautifully above the water. Most people recognize the flowers, usually pink or rosy and sometimes white. The flower symbolizes birth, creation, and reproduction, and it has been one of the most important symbols in Asian culture. Where most plants become fruit after the flowers wither, the lotus plant blooms its flowers and its fruit simultaneously, symbolizing birth and creation.

Sacred lotus also symbolizes honesty, beauty, and virtue. The lotus flower shows the beauty in our different backgrounds. Whether we were born rich or poor, beauty is seen when you look into the depths of a person's soul. The lotus flower is grown in muddy and dirty waters, yet the beauty attracts all people because it makes no pretense of being better than it is. Many people see the price in beauty by what a person wears, their bodily figure, and their face painted with makeup, but a few people see the value in natural beauty—bare soft skin, wrinkles from the laughter and tears throughout the years, and strands of gray and white hairs symbolizing wisdom. The soul is meant to wear a crown of light and dignity.

The flower essence of the lotus is an excellent way for enhancing and harmonizing higher consciousness and acts as a spiritual elixir or harmonizer. In Confucianism and Buddhism, it is depicted as one who has overcome the pains of the material world and becomes enlightened.

The beautiful lotus flower grows in murky water but manages to surpass the muddy conditions and produce an enchanting flower that is praised among many cultures and religions. Similar to us, when the evening approaches the flower bud closes, ready for bed, and in the morning, the lotus blossoms with a pure heart, open to new beginnings. Rest is necessary for our bodies to restore and regenerate, giving us more clarity and energy for a new day.

recipe follows

BRAISED LOTUS ROOT

찐 연꽃 [jjin yeonkot]

The crunchy root of the pond flower is mild in flavor and tastes like a combination of a potato and radish. Cylindrical and brown, its lacelike design looks like a rooted snowflake. This is a simple snack that's great with a bed of rice and seaweed.

SERVES 4 TO 6

1 pound (455 g) lotus
  root, peeled and sliced
  in ¼-inch (6 mm) slices
1 tablespoon (15 ml)
  vinegar
1 cup (235 ml) water
4½ tablespoons (68 ml)
  soy sauce
2 tablespoons (28 ml)
  rice wine
1½ tablespoons (23 g)
  packed brown sugar
1 tablespoon (15 ml)
  olive oil
2 tablespoons (28 ml) rice
  malt syrup
½ tablespoon sesame oil
½ teaspoon sesame seeds,
  for garnish

1. In a medium-sized pot, add the lotus root with enough water to cover. Add the vinegar and cook for 10 to 15 minutes, depending on how soft you would like to eat the lotus root. Drain and rinse with cold water.

2. To braise: Return the slices to the pot and add the water, soy sauce, rice wine, brown sugar, and olive oil. Bring to a boil, uncovered, over medium-high heat for 15 to 20 minutes until the liquid is reduced to about ¼ cup (60 ml). Stir occasionally to evenly cook the lotus root slices.

3. Add the rice malt syrup and sesame oil and then stir for 3 to 4 minutes. Garnish with sesame seeds to serve.

—

I find joy in the midst of anger, sorrow, or pain.

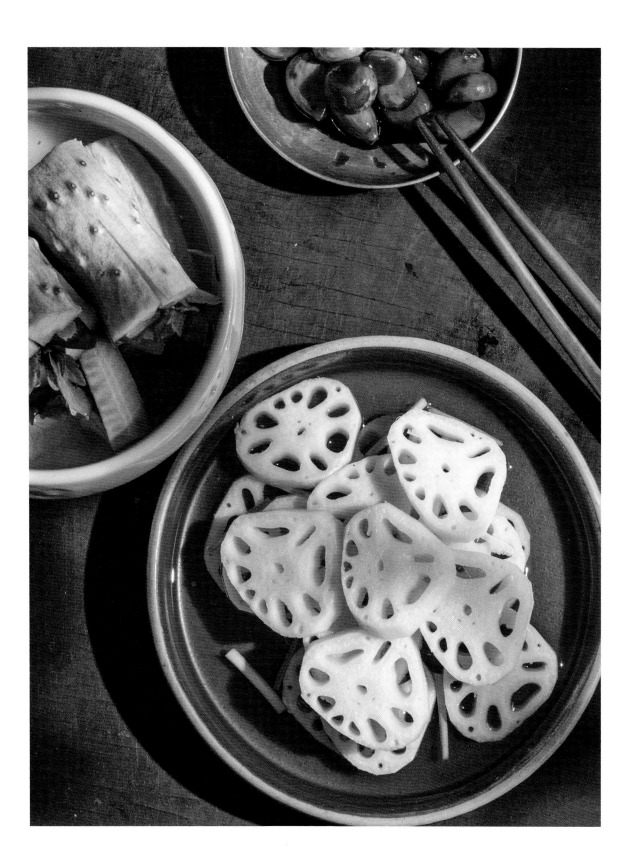

Skullcap 골무 꽃 [golmu-kott]

FAMILY: Labiatae

GENUS: *Scutellaria baicalensis*

COMMON NAMES: Baikal skullcap, Huang Qin, blue skullcap

PART USED: root

EFFECTIVE QUALITIES: cold and dry, bitter, astringent, relaxant, vital stimulant

NATIVE REGIONS: Korea, China, Mongolia, Russia

CONSTITUENTS: bitter (iridoids), flavonoids, volatile oil, resin, tannins (rosmarinic acid), essential oils, fixed oil

PROPERTIES: antioxidant, anti-inflammatory, anticonvulsant, sedative, uterine relaxant, laxative, choleretic, nervine tonic, hypnotic, lowering attributes

INDICATED USES: fever, inflammation, common cold, jaundice, dysentery, diarrhea

NUTRIENTS: iron, zinc, calcium, magnesium phosphate, potassium sulfate, chlorophyll

—

PREPARATION: Skullcap is prepared fresh or dried by long infusion or tincture.

DOSE: Long infusion: 8–10 grams; tincture: 2–4 milliliters at 1:3 strength in 45 percent ethanol

CAUTION: Skullcap supplements have been found adulterated with germander, a toxic herb, so make sure you are carefully sourcing this herb. It may also interact with certain medications, so consult with your Eastern medical practitioner or healthcare provider before use.

—

Skullcap has square stems in a cross section, several arising from the base. The leaves are long and wide, and the flowers bloom in a cluster. The Eastern version of skullcap is the opposite of the common skullcap herb in the West called *Scutellaria lateriflora*. So it is important to recognize the Latin names of herbs since there is more than one herb called skullcap. Baikal skullcap is used in Eastern medicine for a draining effect and for clearing heat. Its main application is for infectious damp-heat conditions.

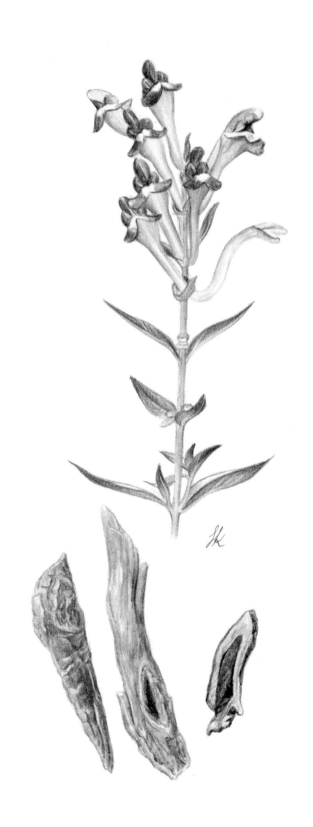

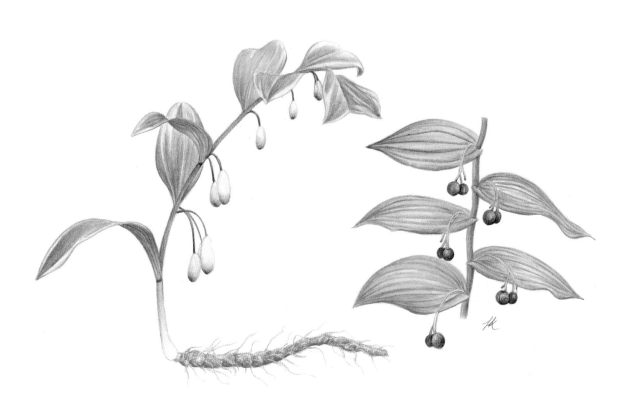

Solomon's Seal
둥굴레 [dong geul lae]

FAMILY: Asparagaceae

GENUS: *Polygonatum odoratum*

COMMON NAMES: King Solomon's seal, Lady's seal

PART USED: rhizome

EFFECTIVE QUALITIES: sweet, moist, restoring, dissolving, relaxing

NATIVE REGIONS: Korea, Japan, China in meadows and sparse woods in lowlands and foothills

CONSTITUENTS: mucilage, tannins, essential oils, saccharides, saponins

PROPERTIES: antitussive, demulcent, diuretic, hypoglycemic, sedative, resolvent

INDICATED USES: convalescence, weakness, febrile diseases

NUTRIENTS: potassium oxalate, trace minerals

—

PREPARATION: Solomon's seal is prepared in decoction or tincture form as well as tea. Topical application is used as a compress to soften and soothe skin and scar tissue.

DOSE: Decoction: 10–15 grams; tincture: 2–5 milliliters at 1:2 strength in 20 percent ethanol

CAUTION: Larger doses and prolonged use of Solomon's seal is contraindicated with intestinal damp and may cause poor digestion, nausea, and diarrhea.

—

How do we gain wisdom? Solomon's seal derives its name from King Solomon, who was known for his wisdom and wealth. The rhizomes from Solomon's seal show the jointed and angled way of life that's not always linear. Several legends describe King Solomon's seal as the shape of a knotty rhizome with indentions that resemble scars. Its many scars that stem from the previous year's growth represent the obstacles and challenges that we face through each year. Scars are markers that remind us of certain events that happened in our lives. Our scars may be visible and remind us of the near-death experiences that we may have faced or scars from giving birth. Solomon's seal is symbolic to how our scars can bring us wisdom throughout the years.

The root is also cherished by ancient Taoists for its restorative properties and as a relished wild vegetable. Unlike Western herbalism, Solomon's seal root is an essential remedy in Eastern herbal practice. With its sweet taste and high content of saponins, Solomon's seal is a nutritive demulcent for treating conditions of yin deficiency with dryness. Similar to asparagus root, Solomon's seal also treats kidney Qi stagnation. It also soothes and protects swollen ligaments and tissue. Besides Solomon's seal being a good bronchial demulcent, it is commonly enjoyed simply as an herbal tea to relax our heart.

Chive 부추 [buchu]

FAMILY: Amaryllidaceae

GENUS: *Allium schoenoprasum*

COMMON NAME: chives

PART USED: herb

NATIVE REGION: worldwide

EFFECTIVE QUALITIES: mild, sweet, somewhat salty, aromatic

CONSTITUENTS: nonvolatile sulfur compounds, saponins, free amino acids

PROPERTIES: cholesterol and triglyceride reducing, antihypertensive, antibacterial, antifungal

INDICATED USES: mainly used as a spice for culinary purposes

NUTRIENTS: vitamin C

—

PREPARATION: Chives are a warming herb and are known to strengthen the intestines. It is great for people who have poor circulation and are constantly cold. Decocting the herb with licorice is an easy way to make an herbaceous chive tea sweetened with licorice. It also helps with postpartum pain.

DOSE: 1–3 grams

CAUTION: Excessive amounts may cause gastrointestinal discomfort.

—

Once native to Asia, chives grow like wildfire and are now cultivated globally. It is one of the most versatile herbs and widely accessible at markets—and can be easy to find in nature if you look closely enough. As a perennial herb, the leaves sprout from the bulb every spring, forming a soft linear shape. In the summer, stems extend between the leaves and small white flowers bloom at the end of the stems.

Growing up, our family would harvest chives from our garden and make Korean chive pancakes or add chives to many of our soups and stews. Harvest young chives that have just broken through soil for the best taste and nutrition content. Chives are rich in protein, and they contain vitamins A and C. The unique scent is due to sulfur compounds that are similar to garlic.

PRAYER TO HEAVEN

As we pray to Heaven, we look to spring and spread our wings for the season to bloom.

We give thanks to Heaven above for the wind and clouds that provide us with air and rain.

Our ancestors are looking down as we pray for blessings and holiness from above.

Remove impurities, selfishness, greed, and deceit so we can truly see beauty and transparency.

Allow the purity of our hearts to transfer to the herbs we create to heal others.

Bring life, healing, and hope.

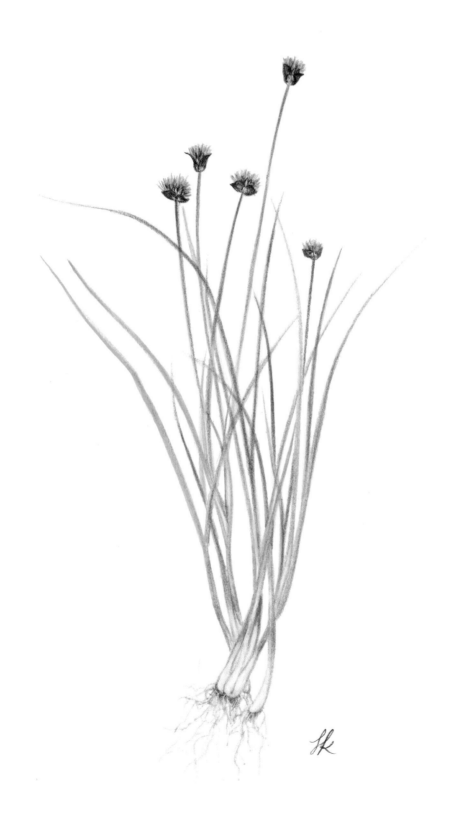

5 | EARTH HERBS OF SUMMER

☷ 곤 [gon]

Umma (mother), salt of the Earth.
Once a daughter, a wife, my mother, and now a grandmother.
Shiny black hair like raven feathers showing her divine nature to nurture and protect.
As the seasons pass, her hair transforms into a dove's wing with strands of silver moon.
She is at peace.
She is our matriarch.

EARTH FOLKTALE: THE TIGER AND PERSIMMON

호랑이와 곶감 [horangiwa gotgam]

In Korea, folktales reflect the enduring culture of our people, thoughts and dreams about nature, and the relationship between humans and nature.

One of my favorite folktales is the "Tiger and Persimmon" because tigers in Korea are a symbol of strength and power and are often seen as a guardian spirit. Aside from persimmons being a favorite sweet treat among Korean people, they are deeply rooted as a Buddhist symbol of transformation—where green bitter fruits transform into bright orange sweet nectar. Persimmons are an important ritual fruit in Korea tracing back to Jongka ancestral rituals, praying to the gods for a rich harvest.

In the middle of the night, a tiger creeps into a village wanting to steal a cow, and coincidentally, a burglar is also attempting to steal a cow. Throughout the night, a child is wailing and crying endlessly. Even when his mother threatens him that a big, scary tiger is coming to eat him, the child keeps crying. Suddenly, the tiger hears the child's mother enticing the child with a persimmon. "Here's a dried persimmon," she says, and then the child stops crying. The tiger is shocked and amused, wondering how dried persimmon has stopped a child from crying. The tiger wonders if the persimmon is more frightening than him as the tiger couldn't scare the child. At the same time, the burglar, who mistakes the tiger for a cow, jumps on the tiger's back. Out of fear, the tiger bolts out of the village with the burglar on his back thinking it was the frightening dried persimmon.

The moral of the story is that mischief (the tiger) and corruption (the burglar) will not prevail if kindness, like the persimmon tree, is deeply planted in the hearts of people.

Persimmons (pronounced "gam" in Korean) have been consumed and used for treating various ailments for centuries in Eastern medicine, and they are a treasured delicacy in Korean culture. Persimmons contain antioxidants, which help prevent oxidative damage and stress. They are great for helping maintain healthy eyes due to high levels of beta-carotene, a vital nutrient for vision and cell growth.

Persimmon 감 [gam]

FAMILY: Ebenaceae

GENUS: *Diospyros kaki*

COMMON NAMES: Sharon fruit, kaki

PARTS USED: fruit, leaves

EFFECTIVE QUALITIES: sweet, mild, rich

NATIVE REGION: East Asia

CONSTITUENTS: folate, phosphorus, calcium, phytochemicals, flavonoid oligomers, tannins, phenolic acids, carotenoids

PROPERTIES: anthelmintic, antihemorrhagic, antitussive, astringent, laxative, expectorant, restorative, antioxidant

INDICATED USES: constipation, diarrhea, coughs

NUTRIENTS: vitamins A, C, and B, potassium, manganese, high in beta-carotene, which lowers the risk of heart disease and certain cancers

—

PREPARATION: Persimmons are commonly consumed as a dessert fruit. The calyx (the outer covering of the fruit) is used for medicinal purposes. Fresh persimmon juice is also used to lower blood pressure.

DOSE: Decoction: 4–8 grams

CAUTION: Persimmons should be consumed in moderation as some individuals may exhibit symptoms of nausea or upset stomach or itchy skin. Make sure to carve out the white flesh underneath the stem to avoid constipation. There are no contraindications when taking persimmon calyx.

—

Eating with the seasons is the best way to enjoy the flavor of fresh herbs and fruits. Crops that are harvested at their peak ripeness are often full of flavor. Not only are fruits and vegetables fresh when picked in season, but they often contain more nutrients as well. To best enjoy the benefits of persimmons, eat them during the fall season. Persimmons can be found at grocery stores and farmers' markets, or if you live on the West Coast, you may be able to stop by a persimmon orchard!

How to Pick a Perfect Persimmon

Picking the perfect persimmon takes some practice, starting with distinguishing between the three varieties of persimmons. All are nutrient dense, but each has a different texture, size, and taste.

Dan-gam (Fuyu, 단감) are yellow-orange in color and shaped like tomatoes. These are the nonastringent type and taste sweet. Dan-gam are great for adding into salads or dried in slices for a healthy snack. The fruit is firm and should soften a bit and has a crispy crunchy taste of fruit.

Hongsi (soft persimmon, 홍시) is sweet, soft, and squishy with paper-thin skin. It has a pureelike texture and is used as a sweetener for baking or cooking. When shopping for either variety of persimmons, choose fruit that are plump but not too firm, with bright orange–colored skin that's free from blemishes. When feelings of worry reside, persimmons will provide nourishment and comfort.

Shaped like large orange-red acorns, Daebong-gam (Hachiya, 대봉감) are astringent and are often dried into gotgam (곶감), also known as hosigaki in Japan. Timing is important in making dried persimmons because the moment a Daebong-gam is at the perfect level of ripeness for drying can quickly pass and then it may turn too ripe and mushy for drying. If you dry it too early, the unripe flesh will create a bitter, chalky taste in your mouth. Similar to the timing in life, there is a certain time of ripeness and opportunity that may quickly pass if we are not mindful of our surroundings.

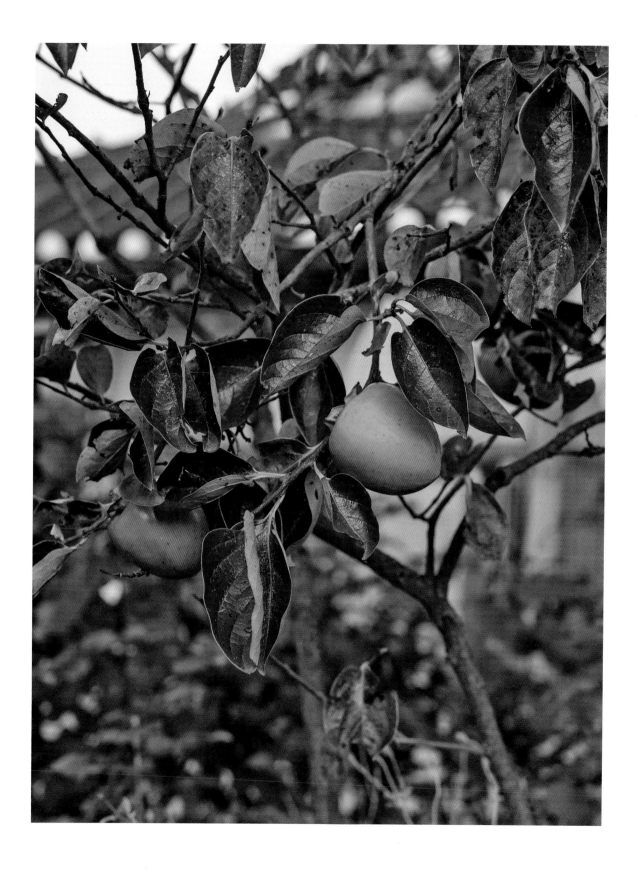

PERSIMMON LEAF TEA

감잎차 [gamipcha]

Makes 4 cups (946 ml) of tea

5 to 6 fresh persimmon leaves or 4 teaspoons (3 g) dried persimmon leaves
4 cups (946 ml) water

One of my favorite leaves to pick on my farm are persimmon leaves. Persimmon leaves contain proanthocyanidins, which are a type of polyphenols, tannins, flavonoids, terpenoids, nitric oxide, choline, astragalin, and amino acids. The leaves also have more vitamin C than the fruit and are a good source of carotenoids, magnesium, manganese, titanium, calcium, and phosphorus. Studies have shown that drinking persimmon leaf tea improves your metabolism, and flavonoids help lower blood pressure. Whenever I see a persimmon tree, I'm reminded of the kindness and nutritious, sweet fruit it bears.

1. To make tea with fresh leaves: Clean and wash the leaves thoroughly. Boil the water and brew for about 10 to 15 minutes.

2. To make tea with dried leaves: Boil the water, add the dried leaves, and brew for about 10 to 15 minutes.

—

The contours of our heart reveals our true intentions.

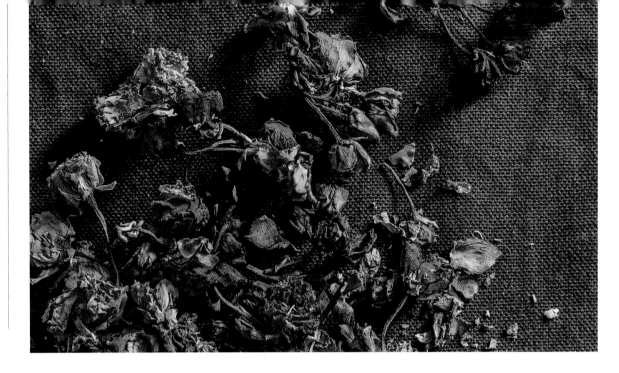

Flower Wisdom

Umma would go to our local flower shop every Saturday to make a ceremonial bouquet. I always wondered if she had memories of her time being a florist when she first came to America. Appa was still in school. Umma said flowers are wise, and there is deep wisdom in giving flowers. We give flowers during many ceremonies, from birthdays to weddings and funerals.

FLOWER ESSENCES

꽃 에센스 [cote esenseu]

TOOLS
Scissors
Crystal bowl
Filtered water
Tweezers
Brandy

One of my favorite ways to give flowers to people I love is by making flower essences. Flower essences are gentle botanical medicine made by imprinting the flowering parts of plants and trees into spring water. The dew from flowers is transformative and healing and brings floral wisdom.

1. Making flower essences is ceremonial. When we approach a flower to harvest, we need to pay homage to the land and greet the flower with our presence. We ask for permission to create medicine. Usually, a gentle breeze or a bird singing are signals that we are allowed to harvest.

2. We give an offering to the place we are planning to harvest. It can be a wide range of offerings from pouring water, singing a song, or giving a strand of hair—whatever feels important to you. I usually sing a song while pouring water to the roots.

3. With scissors, clip right below the flowerhead. Water holds an imprint, so we place the flowerheads over water and begin the solar infusion process. This lasts at least 4 hours, usually between 10 a.m. and 2 p.m. as the sun is at its peak. During the infusion process, we can sit with the plant in quietness or go for a hike, journal, or sit under a tree. I tend to sit with the flowers in quiet reverence.

4. The elements of earth, air, fire, water, and sun are happening during the infusion process. As herbal alchemists, our gardens are considered our laboratory of nature, and the elements earth, air, fire, water, and sun are in harmonious balance. We harvest and gather fresh, dew-filled blooms on a clear, sunny day. Allow the blooms to float in a bowl of pure and filtered water as they absorb the sun's light and warmth for several hours. The process creates an energetic imprint in the water, integrating the healing essence of the flower.

5. Essences are multifaceted, so in choosing a flower essence, we look to the cardinal directions: North for tradition, South for personal experience, East for knowledge, and West for intuition. The cardinal directions will reveal what areas in our life we need to heal and grow. If we are conflicted with certain traditions that we grew up with, we ask the North to give us more clarity and appreciation for the tradition. If we are experiencing a personal challenge that was from our past or we are currently facing, we ask the South for peace and forgiveness. If we are planning to make a major life decision, we ask the East for wisdom and guidance. If we are faced with uncertainty, we ask the West to strengthen our intuition and really listen to our inner voice.

6. Across cultures, flowers show us the blossoming of our spirit. Every flower has a distinct personality and gift in healing us. When emotions of sadness, fear, anger, pain, and depression are stuck in our body, flower essences are a beautiful way of helping us move stuck energy.

7. As we sit with our flower essence in prayer, we say our name as it was given to us—a gift of life. Then, we take a few drops under our tongue and pause for a moment, closing our eyes and thanking the universe for giving us this one precious life. Whatever we are going through, we are close to Mother Earth as she provided us with our flower essence to help protect us, guide us, and grant us peace.

—

Floral meanings: Lily: Purity of heart; Magnolia: Dignity of yin; Azalea: Remembrance of first loves; Daffodil: Truth and mercy; Chrysanthemum: Strong friendship; Sunflower: Loyalty in relationships

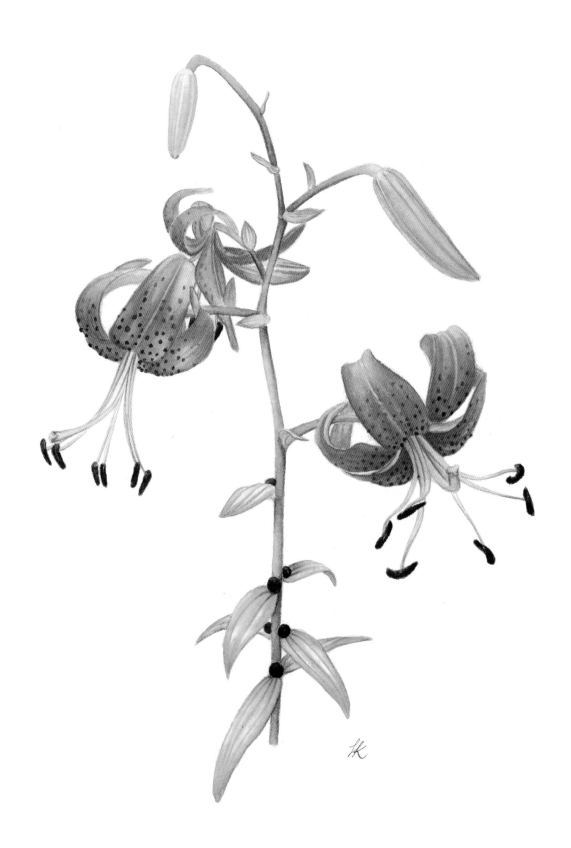

Tiger Lily 참나리 [chamnari]

FAMILY: Liliaceae

GENUS: *Lilium lancifolium*

PART USED: tuber

EFFECTIVE QUALITIES: cough, sore throat, palpitation, boils

NATIVE REGIONS: Korea, Guam, China, Japan

CONSTITUENTS: essential oils, mucilage, mildly alkaline, mildly acid

PROPERTIES: anti-inflammatory, diuretic, emmenagogue, emollient, expectorant

INDICATED USES: balances out overly aggressive yang forces or excessive competition

—

PREPARATION: Water infusion of tiger lilies preserved in brandy; lily bulbs are eaten raw or cooked in culinary dishes.

DOSE: Take 5 drops under your tongue 3 times a day every day for a month to help initiate lasting change.

CAUTION: Do not use tiger lily if you have diarrhea or have a cough. It may cause drowsiness. Tiger lilies are highly toxic to cats, so please make sure the flower is kept away from your feline friend.

—

Umma made the most beautiful bouquets, and tiger lilies were one of her favorite flowers. Native to Korea, the tiger lily, a sun-kissed flower with black speckles, is wildly foraged throughout Asia for its edible bulbs. The tiger lily symbolizes protection against harm. Its bold and unique colors ward off evil spirits. This particular species does not produce seeds but instead it produces little black bulbs where the leaves meet the stem.

The tiger lily essence is for self-protection and setting firm boundaries. We tend to overextend ourselves to others and may lose our own identity along the way, so the tiger lily reminds us to shift our priorities and protect our time and energy so we can give more without depleting our energy. The tiger lily is a remedy for helping our soul to transmute aggressive tendencies into positive social impulses. It helps our consciousness to transition from a limited personal perspective toward values that are global.

The tiger lily balances dominant yang energy and is helpful for those who have not fully embraced their inner feminine yin. The flower helps bring peace and harmony into our lives, providing strength to our soul to improve society and the world.

Cool Cucumber Summers

Summers in Texas are like spicy red Korean chile peppers fried in a cast-iron skillet. The sun beating on Grandma's back, a rolling hill extended down to her Korean garden that no one knew except wise women—she brought a piece of Korea with her because she missed her motherland. As a child, I would run down the rolling hill with a glass jar of refreshing cucumber punch because I knew she would never ask for anything, even when she was thirsty.

The only English words Grandma knew were *hi* and *cola*. But she recognized all the presidents' faces on paper currency, especially Benjamin Franklin's. A woman who didn't have a "regular job" always had money to give us, and now I understand why. It was her vast and fruitful garden. People always came to see her and harvest Korean herbs and vegetables to take home to their families. All those dollars she collected and rolled in her pocket she saved for a rainy day. One of her favorite summer drinks was Korean cucumber water, made from pickled cucumber. It is a refreshing and flavorful drink or cold soup.

KOREAN CUCUMBER PUNCH

오이냉국 [oi nenggook]

SERVES 6 TO 8

2 large seedless cucumber, like an English cucumber (about 20 ounces [567 g])
2 cloves garlic, minced
2 teaspoons soy sauce
3 teaspoons brown sugar or honey
8 teaspoons (39 ml) white or brown rice vinegar
3 teaspoons salt
2 cups (475 ml) water
1 cup (217 g) ice

Cucumbers are a typical summer vegetable with a refreshing taste and aroma that is universal to all. Grandma would say that cucumbers grown under intense sunlight are the most nutritious and delicious. They retain a lot of water, cooling down heat in our body and hydrating us. The mildly astringent effect also cleanses our skin and tightens pores. This salty and sour punch recipe will keep us refreshed during the hot summer season.

1. Clean the cucumbers and slice them into fine strips about 3 inches (7.5 cm) long.

2. Place the cucumber strips into a mixing bowl and add the minced garlic.

3. Add the soy sauce, sugar or honey, vinegar, and salt into the bowl and mix all the ingredients until the sugar and salt are dissolved.

4. Add the water and ice into the bowl of cucumbers.

—

Crunch seasons come to us all. We are refreshed by the coolness of oi punch.

Korean Monk's Hood
백부자 [baekbuja]

FAMILY: Ranunculaceae

GENUS: *Aconitum koreanum*

COMMON NAMES: monk's hood, blue rocket, devil's helmet

PART USED: rhizome

EFFECTIVE QUALITIES: mildly acidic, neutral, mildly alkaline

NATIVE REGIONS: East Asia, Korea

CONSTITUENTS: polysaccharides

PROPERTIES: relieves diuresis, cardiotonic, analgesia, neuralgia

INDICATED USES: chills in legs and arms, articular pain, rheumatic and neuralgic pains, gout, eliminates free radicals

NUTRIENTS: N/A; this plant is toxic and should not be ingested.

—

CAUTION: Korean Monk's Hood is very toxic and is not used for self-treatment. Consult with your Eastern medicine practitioner, healthcare provider, or herbalist about using monk's hood.

—

Looks can be deceiving. This tuberous perennial shrub can be found in grassy areas in mountain valleys or on slopes. The beautiful summer blooms in yellow and light purple may look innocent, but its roots are poisonous. The roots contain highly toxic alkaloids and can cause hypotension and arrhythmia.

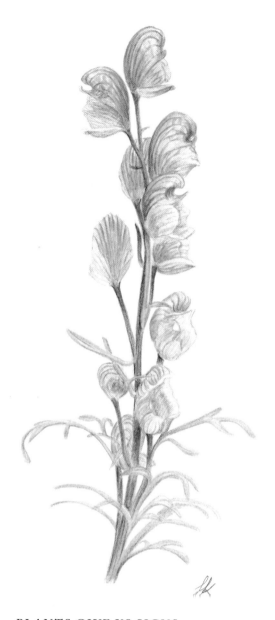

PLANTS GIVE US SIGNS

As time goes by, the simple truth about plants is that they are here to teach us life lessons. Leaves have various geometric shapes—oval, linear, palmate, elliptical. Their arrangements are simple or compound. When a particular herb comes into our life, it fills our hearts with special things that are unexplainable. When we reach for the plant, it is always there to welcome us. We can't measure its worth because once it fills our soul, it is priceless.

Tiger Grass
호랑이풀 [horangipul]

FAMILY: Apiaceae

GENUS: *Centella asiatica*

COMMON NAMES: Centella asiatica, gotu kola, Asiatic pennywort, tiger grass

PART USED: herb

EFFECTIVE QUALITIES: warm and dry, stimulant, tonic, somewhat sweet, bitter, pungent

NATIVE REGIONS: East Asia, Southeast Asia

CONSTITUENTS: saponosides (asiaticoside, madecassoside), flavonoids, phytosterols, carotenoids, skin-soothing agent

PROPERTIES: hypotensive, diuretic, digestive, antiseptic, anti-inflammatory, antioxidant

INDICATED USES: cerebral stimulant and tonic, wound healing, skin issues such as pruritus, psoriasis, boils, and lymphadenitis, reduces inflammation, cellulite, varicose veins, mental and physical fatigue, brightening

NUTRIENTS: vitamin C

—

PREPARATION: Tiger grass can be prepared in many different ways from infusions and tinctures to skin care.

DOSE: Infusions and decoctions: 10–30 grams; tincture: 2–5 milliliters at 1:3 strength in 45 percent ethanol

CAUTION: Tiger grass should not be used during pregnancy and breastfeeding or by individuals with liver disease or epilepsy.

—

Centella asiatica is an ancient plant remedy. People noticed tigers rolling around in this specific grass to heal any infections on their body and started using it for their own skin wounds—hence, the common name tiger grass. It has superlative detoxifying actions and is rich in amino acids, beta-carotene, fatty acids, and phytochemicals. Tiger grass has been used internally and externally. In the beauty industry, it is known to improve skin elasticity and hydrate the skin, offering antiaging effects. Similar to sage or milky oat berry, tiger grass is also an immune restorative and aids in cerebral, nervous deficiencies such as mental and physical fatigue and stress-related disorders.

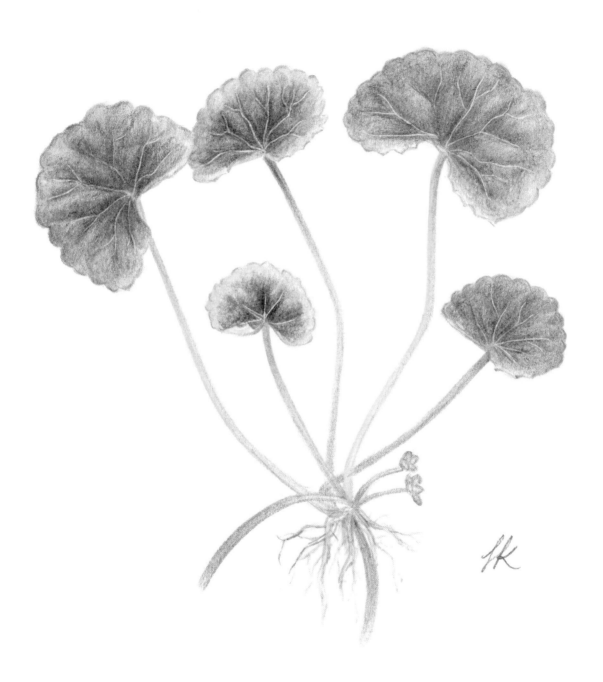

Coltsfoot 머위 [meowi]

FAMILY: Asteraceae

GENUS: *Tussilago farfara*

COMMON NAMES: horsefoot, foalfoot, coughwort, sowfoot

PARTS USED: leaf, flower

EFFECTIVE QUALITIES: bitter, somewhat astringent, pungent, and sweet, restoring, stimulating, decongesting, mucilaginous

NATIVE REGION: Eurasia

CONSTITUENTS: polysaccharides, tannins, flavonoids, coumarins, phenolic acids, minerals

PROPERTIES: demulcent, antitussive, emollient, anti-inflammatory, antibacterial

INDICATED USES: Internally, it is used as a tea or as a culinary dish. Externally, it is used as a mouthwash for mouth and throat inflammation and for skin inflammation.

NUTRIENTS: zinc, vitamin C

—

PREPARATION: Internally, it is used as a tea for inflammation of the upper respiratory tract and as a Korean culinary side dish. Externally, the fresh crushed leaves can be applied in a poultice for topical conditions and also used as a mouthwash for inflammations of the mouth and throat.

DOSE: Infusion: 6–14 grams; tincture: 2–6 milliliters at 1:3 strength in 35 percent ethanol

CAUTION: Coltsfoot should not be used during pregnancy and breastfeeding or by individuals with liver disease, heart disease, or high blood pressure. Coltsfoot contains pyrrolizidine alkaloids and thus should be used externally only.

—

Growing in shady wetlands at the foothills of mountains, coltsfoot leaves look like the hooves of a horse. This is a versatile herb useful for the lung and throat. It is also a great anti-inflammatory. The herb is better applied in lung syndromes that present heat, such as lung phlegm-heat and lung yin deficiency. It is amazing to learn how living processes organize themselves in such complexity to create an herb with significant medicinal properties. We are grateful that such remedies like coltsfoot exist.

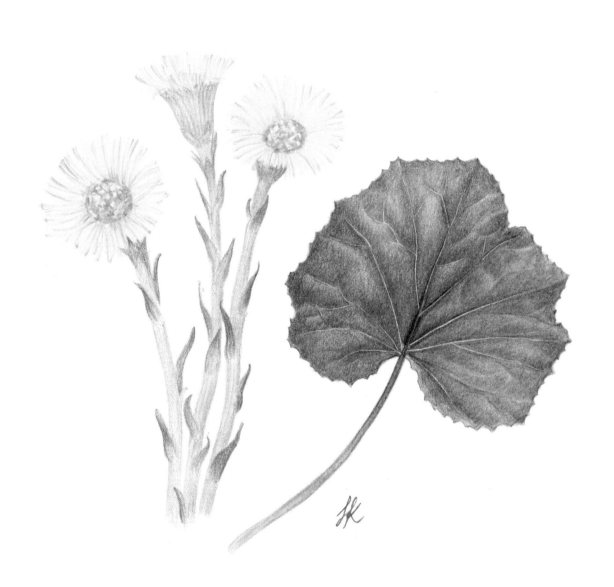

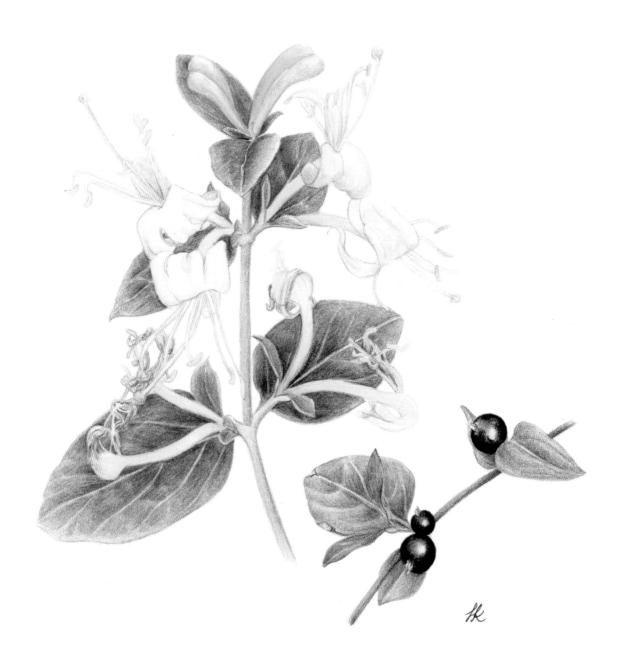

Honeysuckle 인동 [indong]

FAMILY: Caprifoliaceae

GENUS: *Lonicera vesicaria*

COMMON NAME: wild honeysuckle

PART USED: flower

EFFECTIVE QUALITIES: sweet, cooling

NATIVE REGIONS: East Asia, Korea, Japan

CONSTITUENTS: flavonoids, phenolic acids, volatile oil

PROPERTIES: anti-inflammatory, antioxidant, bitter tonic, astringent, diuretic, antiviral, antibacterial, antispasmodic

INDICATED USES: swelling, fevers, inflammation of the upper respiratory tract, minor skin inflammations

NUTRIENTS: vitamins A, B, and C

—

PREPARATION: Internally, the buds are used either raw, dried, or distilled. Externally, it is used as a poultice for minor skin inflammations.

DOSE: Decoction: 5–15 grams; salve: 10–20 grams

CAUTION: There are no contraindications or side effects when used properly.

—

A traditional shrub with flowers used in folk medicine, honeysuckle is rich in flavonoids and phenolic acids. It also contains high antioxidant and antibiotic properties. Honeysuckle buds are gathered in the beginning of summer and then dried in a shaded area. It is consumed as a tea for fevers and inflammatory conditions around the upper respiratory tract. For minor skin inflammations and abrasions, the honeysuckle flowers are made into a poultice and applied to the skin.

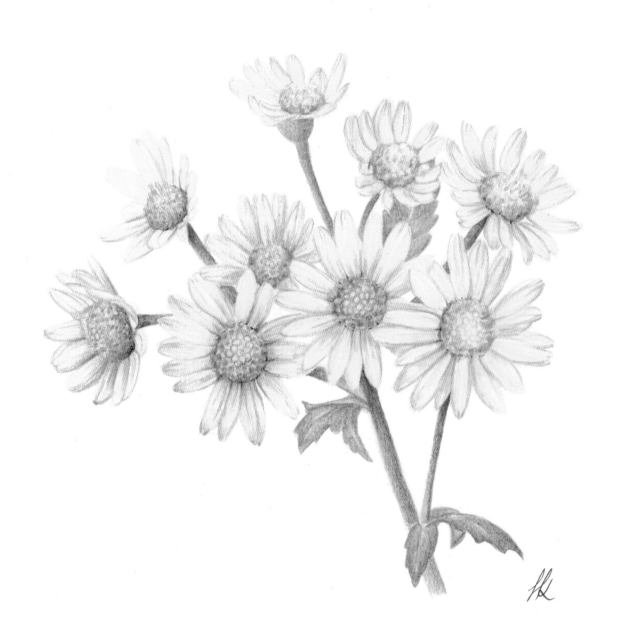

Chrysanthemum
국화 [gukhwa]

FAMILY: Asteraceae

GENUS: *Chrysanthemum indicum*

COMMON NAMES: mums, chrysanths

PART USED: flower

EFFECTIVE QUALITIES: pungent, sweet, bitter, cooling

NATIVE REGION: East Asia

CONSTITUENTS: flavonoids and phenolic acids

PROPERTIES: anti-inflammatory, antibacterial, depurative, febrifuge

INDICATED USES: anxiety, insomnia, congestion, colds, flu, high blood pressure, fever, headache

NUTRIENTS: vitamin B_1, amino acids

—

PREPARATION: Chrysanthemum is commonly taken in tea or tincture form. The leaves and stalks are used in culinary dishes by blanching them in boiling water. Externally, chrysanthemum is used in lotions for skin-care conditions.

DOSE: Infusion or decoction: 5–15 grams

CAUTION: Individuals who are allergic to ragweed should not take chrysanthemum.

—

A member of the daisy family, chrysanthemum flowers have been used in Eastern medicine for thousands of years and are known to help treat a variety of health issues including sleep disorders, anxiety, digestive issues, congestion, high blood pressure, headaches, and fevers. The flowers help expel wind, calm the liver, and clear away heat due to their cooling property. In Eastern medicine, the combination of chrysanthemum and honeysuckle flowers is used to effectively reduce blood pressure.

recipe follows

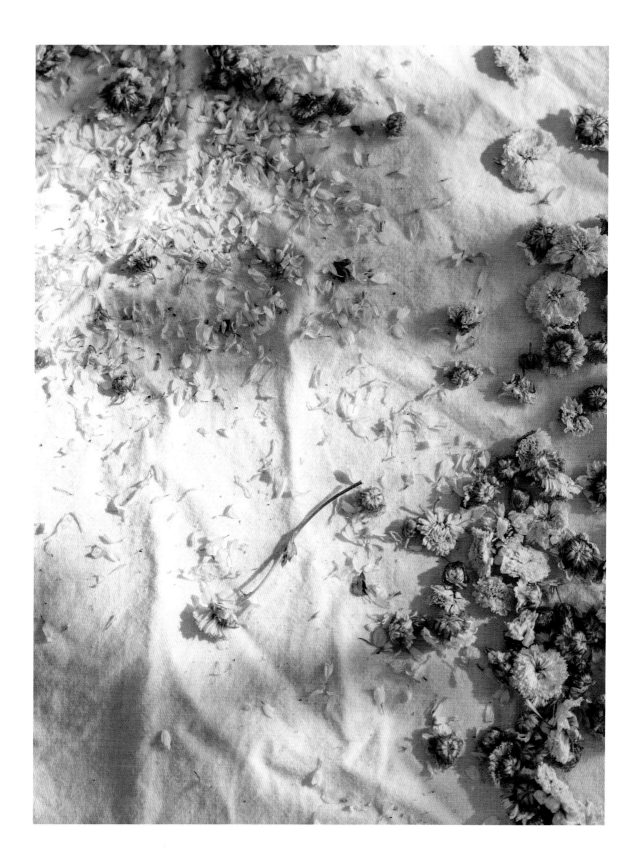

CHRYSANTHEMUM DREAM PILLOW

국화 꿈베개 [gughwa kkumbegae]

Dried chrysanthemum
flowers
Small cotton drawstring
bag

Quality deep sleep is essential for our Qi as it reduces the risk of disease, helps our brain function, balances our emotions, and enhances our dreams. Whenever I have vivid dreams, I draw my chrysanthemum pillow close to my head so I take in the important messages within my dreams. Add other aromatic herbs such as lavender, valerian, rose petals, or chamomile to enhance your dream pillow.

1. Harvest chrysanthemum flowers and dry the flowers in a well-ventilated straw basket or on a window screen in a shaded area for about 2 to 3 weeks. Occasionally shift and rotate the flowers for an even dry.

2. Alternatively, gather the flowers, including the stems. Tie a bunch and hang them upside down in a dry, dark area in a ventilated place, such as an attic, for about 2 to 3 weeks.

3. Fill the drawstring bag with the dried chrysanthemum and secure it tightly.

—

I am the only one holding the power to dream and live a fulfilling life.

Hibiscus 무궁화 [mugunghwa]

FAMILY: Malvaceae

GENUS: *Hibiscus syriacus*

COMMON NAMES: rose of Sharon, althaea

PART USED: bark

EFFECTIVE QUALITIES: antifungal, hypoglycemic, antiulcer, anthelmintic

NATIVE REGIONS: Mauritius, Madagascar, Fiji, Hawaii

CONSTITUENTS: flavonoids, organic acids, phenolic acids, polysaccharides

PROPERTIES: diuretic, acidulous, refrigerant

INDICATED USES: stomach pain, dysentery, omalgia

NUTRIENTS: vitamins C and B, calcium, magnesium, potassium, carbohydrates

—

PREPARATION: Hibiscus is commonly taken in tea form by decocting the flowers in simmering water.

DOSE: Decoction: 10 grams of an infusion with dried calyx

CAUTION: Hibiscus should not be used during pregnancy and breastfeeding. If you have high or low blood pressure or are on medication, consult your Eastern medicine practitioner or healthcare provider before taking hibiscus.

—

The mugunghwa is Korea's national flower as it symbolizes the struggles and victories that the Korean people experienced and endured during wars. Commonly planted in gardens and seen along roadsides, the flower is able to grow resiliently near streets because of its tenacity and fast growth.

One of the most tragic assaults to a woman's dignity is the exploitation and commercialization of her sexuality. The wounds of their souls are deep, and many women feel a disconnect to their sexuality, which should be a warm connection. Often, sexuality is divided from deeper feelings of love and warmth, which come from the heart.

Hibiscus essence helps us to reclaim our sexuality and to restore our Qi with vitality and authenticity. It can aid many people who have been sexually traumatized and is beneficial for all modern people who unconsciously absorb social media images of what beauty means. Hibiscus is also used for those with dominant yang who need to develop a stronger relationship to feminine warmth and positive sexuality. Hibiscus creates flowing warmth throughout the body and soul, especially healing sexuality.

MUGUNGHWA

Mugunghwa, the eternal blossom that never grows faint.
Even during dark and weary days, you are devoted to stay.
Spirit and splendid beauty, you represent Korea.

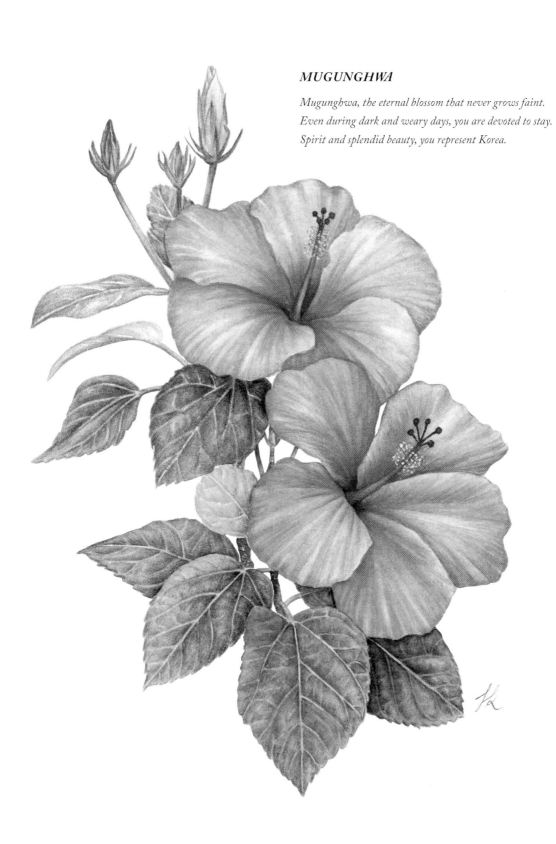

Korean Bramble
복분자 [bokbunja]

FAMILY: Rosaceae

GENUS: *Rubus coreanus*

COMMON NAME: Korean blackberry

PART USED: fruit

EFFECTIVE QUALITIES: polysaccharides, triterpenoids, antioxidant, antipyretic

NATIVE REGIONS: Korea, Japan, China

CONSTITUENTS: minerals, flavonoids, acids, tannins, glycosides, terpenes

PROPERTIES: antioxidant, anticarcinogenic, anti-inflammatory, antimicrobial, antidiabetic, anti-diarrheal, antiviral

INDICATED USES: liver and kidney problems, back pain, tonic, impotence

NUTRIENTS: vitamin A

—

PREPARATION: Korean bramble is used as an herbal medicine by extraction or in a culinary dish. Besides using bramble as a fresh fruit, it is also used as an ingredient in cooked dishes, salads, and bakery products like jams, snacks, desserts, and fruit preserves.

DOSE: 0.5–1 grams

CAUTION: There are no contraindications or side effects when used properly.

A species of raspberry and native to Korea, the Korean bramble is a deciduous prickly shrub that's grown in the thickets of mountain slopes. The stems are purplish red with arching branches.

—

Many studies claim that the fruit reduces the risk of asthma and allergies and helps reduce inflammation. Its dry, astringent quality can relieve mucus discharge, and it is a great anti-inflammatory for throat respiratory issues. Many Koreans enjoy drinking a fruit wine made from fermented Korean bramble berries called bokbunja ju (복분자주), which is known to be an aphrodisiac and a restorative tonic.

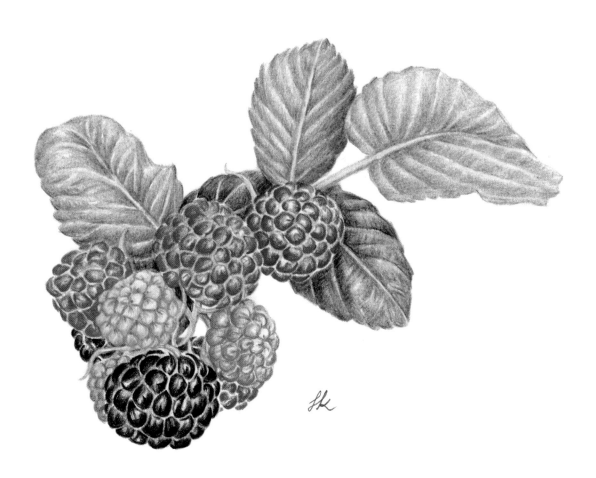

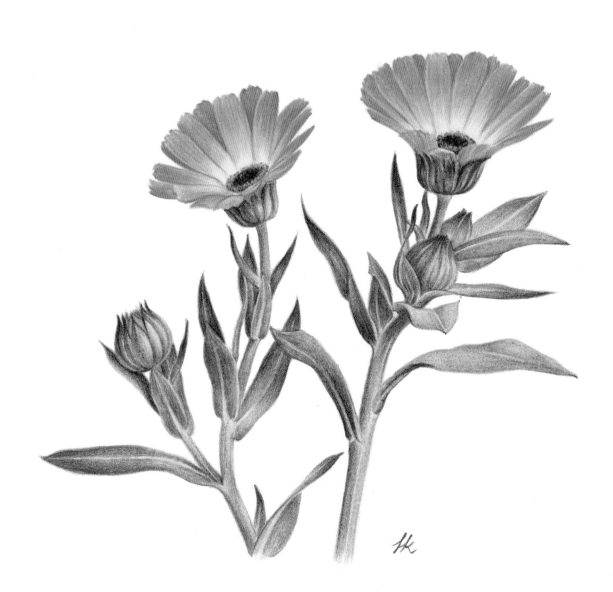

Common Marigold
금잔화 [geumjanhwa]

FAMILY: Asteraceae

GENUS: *Calendula officinalis*

COMMON NAMES: calendula, pot marigold, Mary's gold, gold bloom

PART USED: flower

EFFECTIVE QUALITIES: sweet, somewhat bitter, salty, pungent, decongesting, softening, dissolving, warm, dry, diffusive, vital stimulant, diffusive, relaxant

NATIVE REGIONS: Northern Africa, Europe

CONSTITUENTS: flavonoids, carotenoids, triterpene saponins, essential oil

PROPERTIES: anti-inflammatory, antimicrobial, immunomodulating, vulnerary, mild antispasmodic, mild diaphoretic, antiseptic, antioxidant

INDICATED USES: sore throat, gingivitis, tonsillitis, mouth ulcers, skin health, warming alternative for liver and bowel

NUTRIENTS: vitamin A, lutein, iodine, carotene, manganese

—

PREPARATION: Tea or tincture form

DOSE: Tea: 1–2 teaspoons of marigold combined with 200 milliliters (7 ounces) of boiling water as a tea; tincture: 1–2 milliliters

CAUTION: There are no contraindications or side effects when used properly, but marigold should not be used during pregnancy or if an individual has an allergy to ragweed.

—

Umma says she's drinking the sun every morning when she sips on marigold tea. The beautiful orange and yellow steeped in hot water smells like the garden it was harvested from. The marigold has multiple meanings depending on which region and culture you are in. A garland of marigolds wrapped around Buddha's statue protects it from evil spirits and represents the south-west cardinal direction to attract wealth and success. In Hinduism, the flower brings good luck and prosperity. The marigold is associated with the Virgin Mary in Christian religion, symbolizing joy and piety. The strength of the sun gives marigolds the brightness that lives inside us.

Marigold is a complex remedy for infections on one spectrum and women's health on the other. Its medicinal properties have a detoxicant action that helps with internal inflammatory wind-heat and tissue trauma such as rashes, burns, and itchiness. It is an excellent blood decongestant, and it has astringent properties that aid in blood flow and women's monthly moon cycle. The powerful combination of hormonal balancing and uterine stimulant with blood-decongestant actions, common marigold addresses various Qi liver stagnation and is a comprehensive menstrual remedy.

Astragalus Root
황기 [hwanggi]

FAMILY: Leguminosae

GENUS: *Astragalus membranaceus*

COMMON NAMES: milkvetch, Mongolian milkvetch

PART USED: root

EFFECTIVE QUALITIES: sweet, somewhat warm, dry, restoring, astringing, stabilizing, antihypertensive, diuretic, immunostimulant, antiulcer, uterine stimulant

NATIVE REGION: Northern China

CONSTITUENTS: flavonoids, polysaccharides, amino acids, saponins, trace minerals

PROPERTIES: immune enhancement, adaptogen, astringent, liver protectant, diuretic, antipyretic, haematic

INDICATED USES: Qi tonic, energy-giving, night sweats, blood tonic, immune stimulant, astringent to gut and pores

NUTRIENTS: fatty acids, amino acids, folic acid

—

PREPARATION: Astragalus root is commonly used as a decoction or tincture. The root is boiled in water and then brewed as a tea.

DOSE: Decoction: 9–15 grams; tincture: 3–5 milliliters of astragalus tincture three times per day

CAUTION: There are no contraindications or side effects when used properly, but astragalus root should not be used if an individual has any autoimmune diseases.

—

A member of the legume family, this short-pubescent perennial herb has a woody base and pealike flowers. Astragalus has been used in Eastern medicine for centuries to treat weak and deficient conditions involving metabolic dysfunctions. The adaptogenic functions enhance cellular metabolism, making more energy available on a cellular level because of its antioxidant, anti-inflammatory and immune-boosting properties. The flavonoids and amino acids in the root contain properties that are protective and restorative to the liver. The root's constituents are highly water soluble and are used in decoction or tincture form.

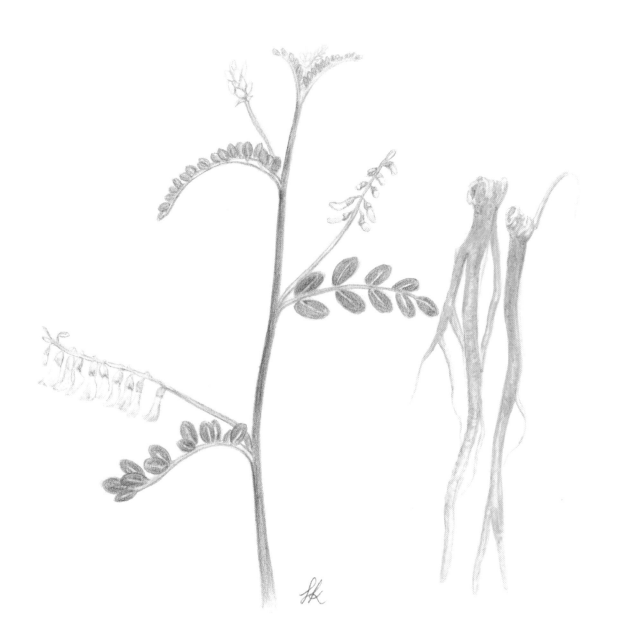

Water Celery 미나리 [minari]

FAMILY: Apiaceae

GENUS: *Oenanthe javanica*

COMMON NAMES: Korean water parsley, water celery, water dropwort, water parsley, Indian pennywort

PART USED: leaf

EFFECTIVE QUALITIES: blood cleanser, liver protectant, lowers blood pressure

NATIVE REGION: East Asia

CONSTITUENTS: persicarin, isorhamnetin, flavonoids, coumarins

PROPERTIES: immune enhancement, ethanol elimination, antioxidant, antiviral, neuroprotective, anticoagulant, anti-fatigue, hypoglycemic, cardiovascular protection, analgesic, insecticidal

INDICATED USES: various chronic and acute hepatitis, jaundice, alcohol hangovers, abdominal pain, inflammatory conditions

NUTRIENTS: vitamins A, B, and C, iron, calcium, potassium, phosphorus

—

PREPARATION: Minari is commonly prepared in culinary form especially in soups, stews, and salads. It is also consumed as tea.

DOSE: 50 grams in culinary dishes

CAUTION: Be extremely cautious when foraging for water celery as it is often mistaken for *Oenanthe crocata*, hemlock water dropwort, which is very poisonous.

—

Minari grows wild along rice fields, streams, and ponds, and it has been cultivated in Asia for thousands of years. It has been used for both food and folk medicine to treat a wide spectrum of diseases. Minari is used in many culinary dishes in Korea and is known for its fibrous roots and aromatic leaves that contain high nutritional value.

MINARI NAMUL SALAD

미나리 나물 [minari namul]

SERVES 6

1 bunch (10½ ounces, or 300 g) water celery
1 tablespoon (15 ml) soy sauce
1 teaspoon chopped scallions
1 teaspoon minced garlic
1 teaspoon honey or brown sugar
1 teaspoon sesame oil
1 teaspoon sesame seeds

A common way to eat minari is making namul, a seasoned herbal side dish. Here is an easy recipe that you can enjoy with rice.

1. Clean the water celery. Remove the leaves and cut the roots. Fill a medium saucepot with salted water and bring it to a boil over medium-high heat. Blanch the water celery for 1 minute and then immediately immerse the water celery in cold water.

2. Rinse, drain, and squeeze out the water. Cut the water celery into 2- to 3-inch (5 to 6 cm) lengths.

3. Add the soy sauce, scallions, garlic, and brown sugar. Massage it into the water celery and mix well. Add the sesame oil and sesame seeds and mix again.

—

A different starting point leads me to the possibilities of change.

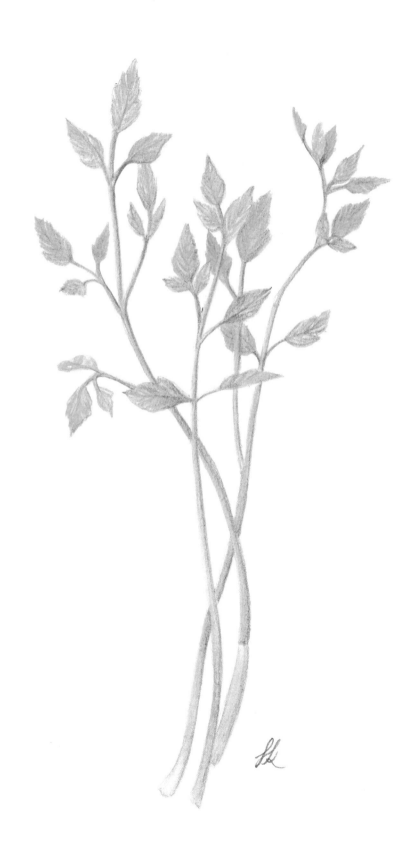

SUMMER MONSOON

Summer monsoon season begins during June or July in Korea, where rain is pouring down. We call this the fifth season, or jang ma. Grandma would mention Korea's monsoon season and would wish for rain to fall in the hot, dry Texas heat. During the summer drifting, masses of moist air move inland from the Pacific Ocean, and as the season changes, we remind ourselves that summer is in constant flux depending on nature's changing course.

Rain cools the earth and gives us freshwater. It feeds our rivers and lakes and keeps plants alive. Rainwater is vital for Mother Nature and plays a magnificent part of balancing the ecosystem.

As a raindrop hits the surface of the earth, it then descends into the ground and becomes groundwater—a vital system for drinking water. Found underground in between cracks in soil and rock, groundwater keeps our rivers flowing. We rely on groundwater for irrigation and drinking water for livestock, and for many rural areas it is the only available option for fresh drinking water. Now when we see a tiny raindrop, we have a different view of how a single drop impacts our lives.

During monsoon season, we make Korean pancakes (see page 160 for the Mung Bean Pancakes recipe) as a tradition. The sizzling sound of the pancakes reminds us of raindrops and how rain is necessary for our plants and ecosystem to thrive.

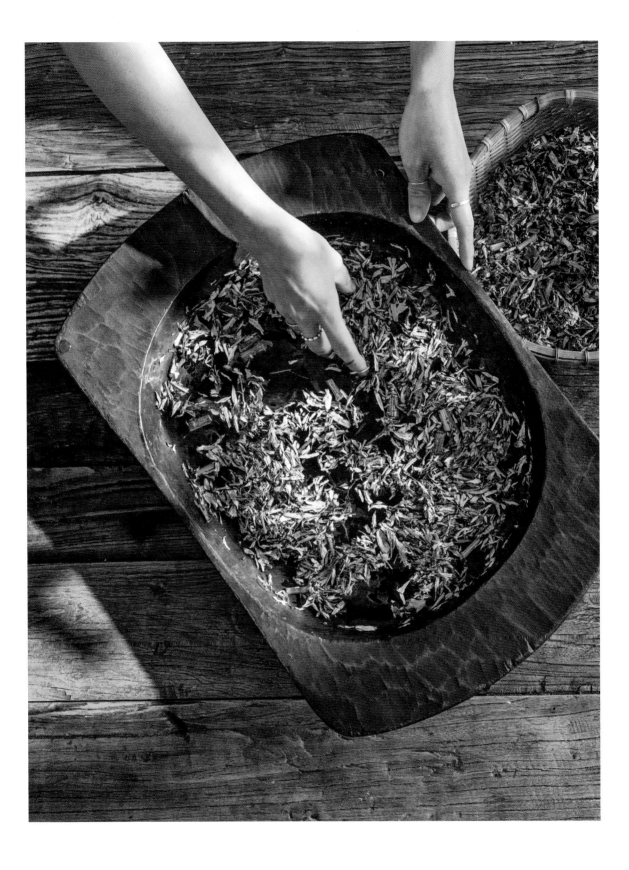

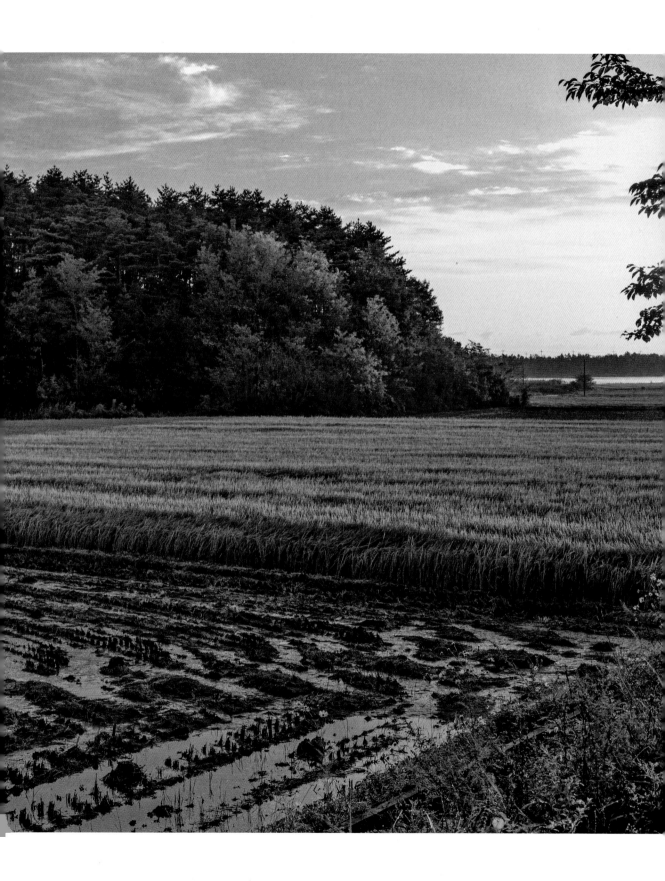

6 SUN HERBS OF AUTUMN

ㅌ 리 [Lee]

Autumn leaves turn red and gold as sisters start to spin like sundown angels.
Never looking back to where we'd been, oh sisters, we hold hands and love with tenderness.
A sister's bond is deep-rooted like a tree bearing sweet fruit.
Her love surrounds you, protects you, and watches over you.

In the mountains of Korea, abundant oak trees produce acorns each autumn and are a viable source of food. Food shortages and famine were common in villages during the first war of the Joseon dynasty in the 1500s, so people foraged the mountains and collected acorns to make dottori-muk (도토리묵), acorn jelly, when grains were unavailable. King Seonjo often ate acorn jelly in remembrance of the hardships during war. As Grandma slowly churned the acorn flour into jelly, tears rolled down her face—memories of famine and the Korean War were her past. Now, her present is in America, the land of the free.

Acorn 도토리 [dotoli]

FAMILY: Fagaceae

GENUS: *Quercus alba*

COMMON NAMES: white oak, English oak, Tanner's oak

PARTS USED: seed, inner bark

EFFECTIVE QUALITIES: very astringent, cool, dry, restoring

NATIVE REGION: Northern Hemisphere

CONSTITUENTS: tannic acids

PROPERTIES: digestive, restorative

INDICATED USES: heart protector, digestion, blood sugar level regulation, bone health, skin care

NUTRIENTS: vitamins A, E, and B, magnesium, folate, calcium, zinc, potassium, iron

—

PREPARATION: The bark is used in decoction and tincture form. The seed is used for culinary purposes.

DOSE: Decoction: 2–6 grams; tincture: 0.5–2 milliliters (10 to 50 drops) at 1:2 strength in 30 percent ethanol

CAUTION: The bark should not be used by individuals with acute diarrhea, constipation, cold symptoms, or kidney or liver disease.

—

The acorns of white oak trees have a number of health benefits that protect the heart, improve digestion, and regulate blood sugar levels. They are a great source of protein and healthy fats, helping to build strong bones, soothe inflammation, and enhance skin care. Acorns have high amounts of tannins, so it is necessary to leach out the tannins before consumption by boiling or soaking. Our ancestors foraged acorns in the mountains for the next generation to nourish on healing foods from Mother Nature.

ACORN FLOUR

도토리 밀가루 [dotoli milgaru]

1 quart (946 ml) acorns

Making acorn flour from foraging your own acorns is a time-consuming but rewarding process as you will taste the fruits of your labor.

1. Collect at least 1 quart (946 ml) of acorns. Sort through the foraged acorns and discard any cracked acorns. Rinse and clean them with water and add them to a bowl. Soak the acorns for 15 minutes and then discard any acorns that remain floating.

2. Next, dry the acorns on a kitchen towel and lay them out on a woven bamboo tray, sheet pan, or window screen. Sun-dry the acorns for at least 2 days and up to 5 days.

3. Once the acorns are dried, crack open the shells with a mallet. Take out the acorn meat and place it in a bowl of water and let it soak in cold water overnight.

4. The following morning, drain the water and replace it with fresh cold water. Do this seven times for seven consecutive days until the water becomes clear. If the acorn meat tastes bland without any bitter taste, then it is ready to be processed.

5. Dry the acorn meat and spread it out on a sheet pan. Preheat the oven to 175°F (80°C). Toast the acorn meat for 90 minutes.

6. Transfer the acorn meat into a food processor and grind it for 45 seconds or until it turns into a powder. Transfer the flour to an airtight container and store it in a cool, dark place. Make sure to avoid direct sunlight.

—

We gather acorns, an important food source for squirrels, in the winter. Let us remember all living beings, not just ourselves.

ACORN JELLY SALAD

SERVES 4 TO 6

ACORN JELLY
½ cup (70 g) acorn flour
3 cups (700 ml) water
½ teaspoon salt

DRESSING
⅓ cup (80 ml) soy sauce
3 cloves garlic, minced
3 scallions, chopped
1 tablespoon (4 g) red
  pepper flakes
2 teaspoons honey
1 tablespoon (15 ml)
  sesame oil

SALAD
½ cup (70 g) acorn flour
8 ounces (225 g)
  chrysanthemum greens
2 cucumbers
7 perilla leaves
1 head lettuce
1 onion
1 bunch Asian chives
2 carrots

도토리묵 샐러드 [dotorimuk saelreodeu]

Acorn jelly is an excellent diet food and helps relieve stomach pains.

1. To make the acorn jelly: In a large bowl, combine the acorn flour, water, and salt. With a wooden spatula, mix and strain the thick liquid to remove any lumps. Pour the mixture into a heavy-bottomed pot and stir over medium heat for 7 to 8 minutes until the mixture bubbles. Lower the heat and stir continuously for 5 minutes. Then, pour the mixture into a glass container. Place the container in the refrigerator to cool for at least 4 hours until it is a solidified jelly. Once the acorn jelly is solid, cut it into cubes and add to the salad mix.

2. To make the dressing: Add the soy sauce, garlic, scallions, red pepper flakes, honey, and sesame oil to a small bowl. Whisk to combine.

3. To make the salad: Thoroughly wash the vegetables. Chop the chrysanthemum greens, cucumbers, perilla leaves, lettuce, onion, chives, and carrots. Add them to a large bowl and toss to combine. Add the cubed acorn jelly and pour in the dressing.

—

Where there are acorns, we smile and share.

SUN FOLKTALE: SISTERS OF THE SEA

We call upon the Haenyo women to tackle the sea and harvest marine life.

For centuries, Jeju, the largest island of South Korea, has been the home to the Haenyo women. This group of free-diving women were the first working women in Korea to make a living harvesting marine life such as shellfish and seaweed. Many of the women support their entire families with their harvest and are true supporters of the ecosystem due to their mindfulness not to overharvest.

Before each harvest, they pray to the sea god for protection and a good harvest. They wrap and toss offerings such as rice or eggs into the sea for an abundant catch and for safety at sea. Haenyo women will continue to live on as a cultural heritage. Through them, I see the strength in my sisters and so many elders that came before us and the sacrifices they made to provide.

Seaweed 미역 [miyeok]

Family: Alariaceae

Genus: *Undaria pinnatifida*

Common names: brown seaweed, sea mustard, wakame

Parts used: leaf, stem

Effective quality: mucilaginous

Native region: East Asia

Constituents: trace minerals

Properties: nutritive, astringent, anti-inflammatory

Indicated uses: supports digestive health, lowers inflammation, increases iron levels in blood

Nutrients: vitamin B_{12}, iodine, iron, magnesium, calcium, potassium, zinc, copper

—

Preparation: decoction, soup

Dose: 4.5 and 15 grams of dried seaweed

Caution: Seaweed counteracts with the properties of licorice root; therefore, seaweed and licorice root should not be taken together. Also, seaweed should be used with caution by patients taking blood-thinning medications.

—

Rich in calcium and iron, seaweed has the same nutritional value as breast milk and is a traditional Korean birthday and postpartum soup for new mothers. Potassium helps lower blood pressure and reduces the risk of heart disease. Seaweed has healing minerals and is high in iodine, which is essential for our metabolism and a healthy thyroid function. While many people assume kelp is a generic name for seaweed, it is not. Kelp is just one type of seaweed often known as kombu.

Not only does seaweed provide nutritional content, it plays an important role in our marine ecosystem and is considered the "forest of the sea." Seaweed produces oxygen and offers shelter for many sea species, so it is important to sustainably farm and harvest to minimally impact our environment.

RESTORATION SEAWEED SOUP

미역국 [miyeogguk]

SERVES 4

1 handful dried kelp
  seaweed
1 teaspoon perilla oil
½ teaspoon chopped
  garlic
1 medium onion
10 mussels, cleaned, or
  ½ pound (227 g) of beef
  tips for a beef broth
1 teaspoon soy sauce
1 teaspoon salt, plus
  more to taste
5 cups (1.2 L) water
Black pepper
Cooked rice, for serving

Every birthday, my mother would make birthday seaweed soup. This Korean tradition will forever be passed on to the next generation as it is a reminder of nourishing a new year of life and longevity.

1. Rinse and soak the seaweed in a large bowl of warm water for 20 minutes or until it becomes rehydrated, moist, and flexible. Drain and cut seaweed into small pieces.

2. In a stockpot, heat the perilla oil over low heat for 2 minutes. Add the garlic, onion, mussels or beef tips, seaweed, soy sauce, and salt. Stir and cook for 5 to 7 minutes over low heat until the onions are softened. The seaweed will turn dark green, turning back into its original fresh color.

3. Add water and boil it over medium-high heat. Lower the heat and simmer the soup for 20 to 30 minutes until the seaweed is soft and tender. Season with salt and pepper to taste. Serve hot with a bowl of rice.

—

To the women of Jeju Island, we give thanks for preserving seaweed and harvesting what we need.

Angelica Dahurica
구릿대 [goo rit dae]

FAMILY: Apiaceae

GENUS: *Angelica dahurica*

COMMON NAMES: garden angelica, dahurian angelica, root of the Holy Ghost

PART USED: root

EFFECTIVE QUALITIES: warm, dry vital stimulant, relaxant, diffusive, pungent

NATIVE REGIONS: Korea, Japan, Northern China

CONSTITUENTS: phytochemicals, ferulic acid, various polysaccharides

PROPERTIES: anti-inflammatory, laxative, sedative

INDICATED USES: headache, toothache, cold, fever, pain

NUTRIENTS: potassium

—

PREPARATION: Decoction or tincture

DOSE: 3–5 grams a day

CAUTION: Angelica dahurica should not be used during pregnancy or by individuals taking certain medications, especially blood thinners. It may also increase the skin's sensitivity to sunlight, and care should be taken when handling as it can cause skin irritation.

—

A member of the Apiaceae family, this perennial herb stands about 3 to 5 feet (91.5 to 152.5 cm) tall and 1 to 2 inches (2 to 5 cm) in diameter, with a stout and hollow stem and short upper branches. Its natural habitat is in wet places near mountain streams.

Warm and pungent in taste, the root has a long medicinal history in Asia. Harvested twice a year in the summer and autumn, its cylindrical roots must be harvested before the stalk emerges. In folk medicine, it plays an important role in dispelling wind, opening up the nasal passages, and curing headaches.

NOTE: Some organic chemical compounds called coumarins activate adrenaline and are the main bioactive constituents in the herb. Coumarins have a spectrum of pharmacological activities that are antiviral, antitumor, and anti-osteoporosis. Studies have also shown that angelica dahurica has more than three hundred chemical constituents ranging from volatile oils, alkaloids, phenols, sterols, polyacetylenes, to polysaccharides.

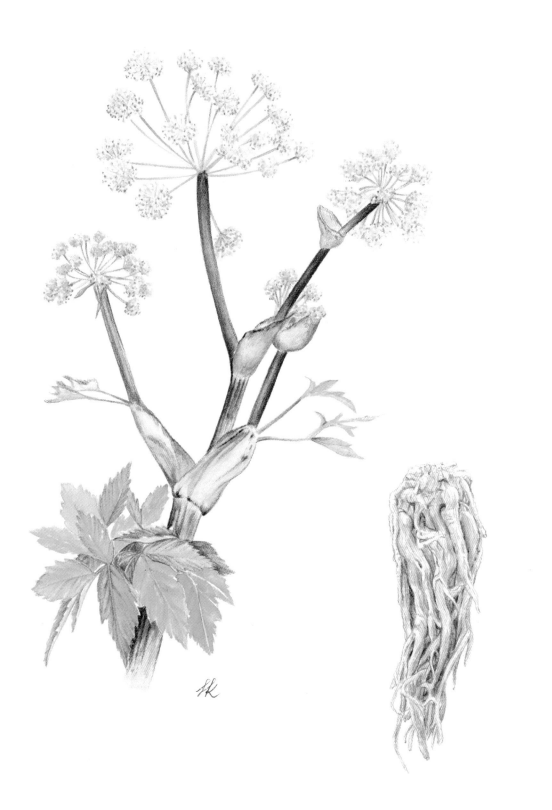

Bellflower 도라지 [doraji]

FAMILY: Campanulaceae

GENUS: *Platycodon gradiflorum*

COMMON NAMES: balloon flower, Korean bellflower, Chinese bellflower

PARTS USED: root, leaves, steams

EFFECTIVE QUALITIES: protects the stomach, reduces inflammation, improves insulin resistance

NATIVE REGION: East Asia

CONSTITUENTS: saponins, flavonoids, phenolic acids, fatty acids, amino acids

PROPERTIES: antitumor, antioxidation, anti-inflammatory, hypoglycemic, anti-obesity

INDICATED USES: reduces inflammation of the upper respiratory tract and gastrointestinal tract, helps relieve hangovers

NUTRIENTS: fiber, potassium, magnesium, phytosterol, betulinic acid, saponins, inulin, glucose, vitamins C and K

—

PREPARATION: Bellflower is taken in culinary, decoction, tincture, or tea form.

DOSE: Tea: 20 grams for 2 liters (2 quarts) of water; decoction: 3–10 grams

CAUTION: Balloon flower should not be used during pregnancy and breastfeeding. Alcohol may interact with the herb.

—

Purple or white bell-shaped flowers bloom vastly in the high mountains and deep valleys throughout Korea from July through August. Before fully blooming, the bud swells like a balloon, hence the common name balloon flower. The five petals are fused together into a bell shape at the base. Its thick roots and stems are about 1 to 3 feet (30.5 to 91.5 cm) tall. Whether dried or fresh, bellflower root is a common herb in traditional Korean cuisine. It has an earthy taste and a crunchy texture with medicinal and anti-inflammatory properties that support the immune system.

recipe follows

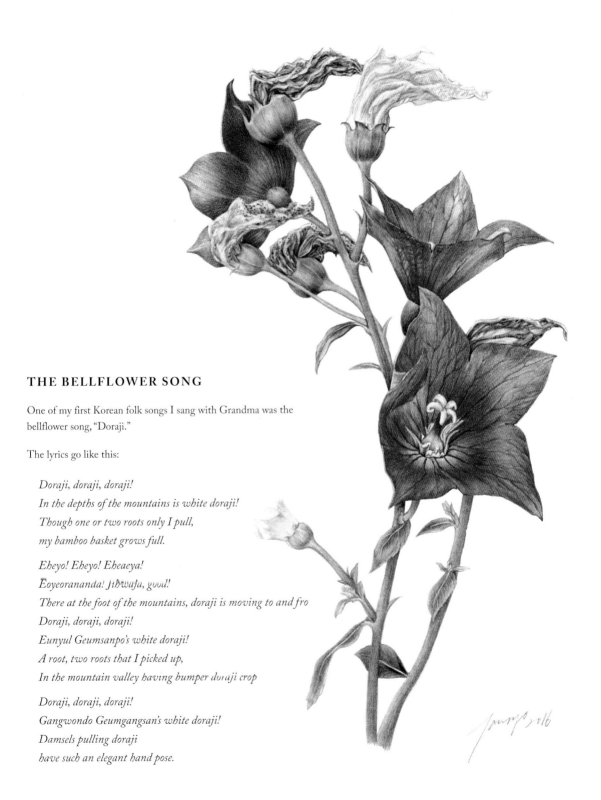

THE BELLFLOWER SONG

One of my first Korean folk songs I sang with Grandma was the bellflower song, "Doraji."

The lyrics go like this:

Doraji, doraji, doraji!
In the depths of the mountains is white doraji!
Though one or two roots only I pull,
my bamboo basket grows full.

Eheyo! Eheyo! Eheaeya!
Eoyeorananda! Jihwaja, good!
There at the foot of the mountains, doraji is moving to and fro
Doraji, doraji, doraji!
Eunyul Geumsanpo's white doraji!
A root, two roots that I picked up,
In the mountain valley having bumper doraji crop

Doraji, doraji, doraji!
Gangwondo Geumgangsan's white doraji!
Damsels pulling doraji
have such an elegant hand pose.

SEASONED BELLFLOWER ROOT

도라지 무침 [doraji muchim]

This is a Korean herbal side dish to go with your daily meal.

SERVES 4

2 tablespoons (32 g) red
    pepper paste
1 teaspoon red pepper
    flakes
1 teaspoon soy sauce
2 tablespoons (28 ml)
    vinegar
1 tablespoon (15 ml)
    brown rice syrup
2⅔ ounces (200 g) whole
    bellflower root, peeled
    and shredded
2 cucumbers, finely
    chopped
1 teaspoon sesame oil
Salt

1. To make the seasoning: Whisk together the red pepper paste, red pepper flakes, soy sauce, vinegar, and brown rice syrup in a small bowl.

2. Add the bellflower root and cucumber to a large bowl. Add the seasoning and toss to combine. Add the sesame oil and toss again to combine. Season to taste with salt and serve.

—

I activate the power of choice by being fully conscious.

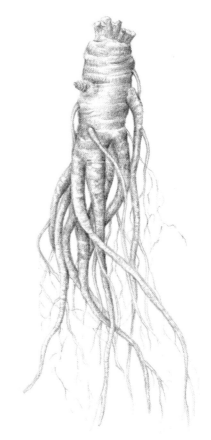

Burdock 우엉 [ueong]

FAMILY: Asteraceae

GENUS: *Arctium lappa*

COMMON NAMES: beggar's buttons, cocklebur, hare lock, bardana, burr seed

PARTS USED: root, seeds

EFFECTIVE QUALITIES: cool and dry, astringent, vital stimulant, somewhat bitter, pungent, dissolving, restoring, stool softener, skin health

NATIVE REGIONS: Asia, Europe

CONSTITUENTS: flavonoids, polysaccharides, bitter glycosides, alkaloid, antibiotic, tannin, resin

PROPERTIES: antibacterial, antifungal, antitussive, diaphoretic, diuretic, emollient, laxative, sedative, alterative, nutritive, bitter tonic, mild hepatic stimulant, antitumor, tonic, demulcent, antiphlogistic

INDICATED USES: constipation, diarrhea, fever, malaria, allergies, rheumatoid arthritis, skin ailments

NUTRIENTS: vitamins B_6 and C, manganese, potassium, folate, calcium, iron, phosphorous

—

PREPARATION: Burdock root is commonly used as a culinary ingredient as well as a tea. Decoction and tincture are also commonly prepared. The fresh root makes the most active antibacterial and antifungal remedy.

DOSE: Decoction: 6–10 grams; tincture: 1–5 milliliters at 1.2 strength in 25 percent ethanol

CAUTION: Burdock should not be used during pregnancy and breastfeeding or by individuals that are taking medicine for diabetes or have an allergy to ragweed.

—

Many underlying issues in our world are being put into question at this time, and there has been a shift in the consciousness about plant remedies. Our healthcare system and big pharma have disappointed us, and we are in search of the root causes of disease, not just another pill that will temporarily relieve our pain. Western society often puts all of its eggs in one basket for curing health issues. There is a pill for everything nowadays. Many Eastern cultures find cures in natural remedies, specifically natural healing herbs that hold medicinal properties like burdock.

Burdock is a perennial plant with coarse stems, large leaves, and purple thistlelike flowers. It is an herb most notable to herbalists and health enthusiasts for its roots. It has a deep taproot that grows up to 6 feet (1.8 m) underground. In the early stages of the plant's life, about one to two years in, all the plant's energy is put into growing the roots of the plant. For this reason, most of the health benefits of burdock are found in the root of the plant while it is young.

Used as a blood purifier, burdock promotes detoxification, reduces lymph congestion, and relieves skin irritations such as eczema. It releases digestive juices and bile, helping with intestinal cleansing, and it is used as a diuretic and digestive aid. It helps to flush out toxins from the body. Burdock has a large amount of antioxidants such as quercetin, luteolin, and phenolic acids. These antioxidants help protect against free radicals, which cause damage to cells.

A lot of issues with skin derive from the liver. Our liver gets overwhelmed working to break down toxins when we eat unhealthy food, and oftentimes, the skin is left to deal with the releasing of toxins because it has pores to let them out. When toxins are released through the skin, we see irritated skin. Burdock clears the liver out, and so with a clean liver comes clear skin. People with regular acne as well as eczema and psoriasis can find solutions in consuming burdock.

recipe follows

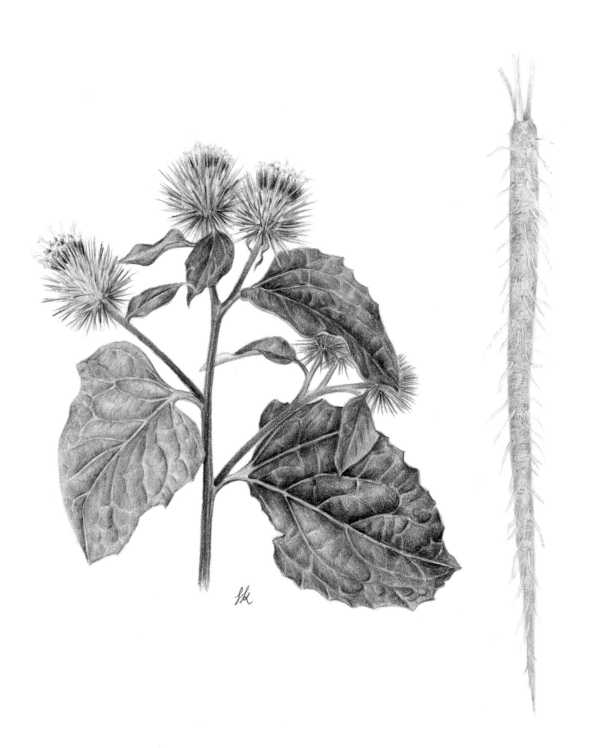

BRAISED BURDOCK ROOT

우엉 조림 [ueong jorim]

SERVES 4

1⅔ cups (200 g) burdock
root, peeled and
julienned
1 tablespoon (15 ml)
sesame oil
1½ tablespoons (25 ml)
soy sauce
3 tablespoons (45 ml)
water
2 tablespoons (28 ml) rice
syrup
¼ teaspoon sesame seeds

Burdock root is a common Korean herbal dish that's an excellent source of fiber and nutrients. The recipe is a delicious way to eat burdock with your meal. I sometimes add braised burdock root to my salads to give them an extra dose of chewiness and sweetness. Everyone needs a little burdock in their life.

1. Bring a pot of water to boil over medium-high heat. Blanch the burdock strips in the boiling water for 3 minutes and then drain in a fine-mesh strainer.

2. Add the sesame oil to a large frying pan and heat it over medium-high heat. Add the burdock strips and stir-fry for 4 to 5 minutes until the burdock is translucent. Add the soy sauce, water, and rice syrup. Simmer over low heat for 8 to 10 minutes. To serve, sprinkle with the sesame seeds.

—

My roots run deep like burdock, protecting me from free radicals and clearing my liver and skin.

❧ BURDOCK TEA

Not only is burdock a great source of protein, it is also a great daily tea to help cleanse our blood.

Take 3 to 4 pieces of dried burdock root (about 1 tablespoon, or 7 g) in 2 cups (475 ml) of hot water and steep it for 20 minutes. This nourishing tea has an earthy and grounding flavor.

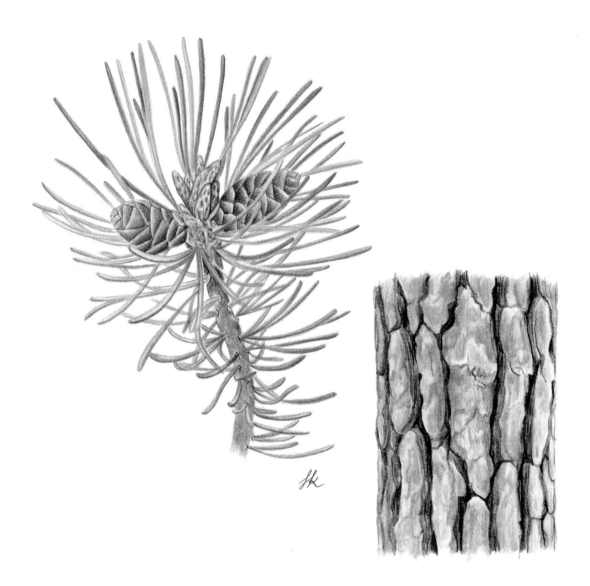

Korean Pine 잣나무 [jatnamu]

FAMILY: Pinaceae

GENUS: *Pinus koraiensis*

PARTS USED: seed, leaves, nuts, bark, and resin

EFFECTIVE QUALITIES: pungent, bitter, aromatic, stimulating, restoring, solidifying, stabilizing

NATIVE REGIONS: East Asia, Korea, Manchuria, Russia

CONSTITUENTS: pinolenic acid

PROPERTIES: antidiabetic agent, galactagogue, analgesic, anti-inflammatory, antibacterial, hypolipidemic, diuretic

INDICATED USES: earache, epistaxis, respiratory complaints, burns, boils

NUTRIENTS: vitamin C, iron

—

PREPARATION: Korean pine nuts are commonly used in culinary form. Decoction or tincture form is also used.

DOSE: Korean pine depends on several factors such as the user's age, health, and other conditions, so please consult with your Eastern medicine practitioner or healthcare provider.

CAUTION: Korean pine nut might cause allergic reactions to individuals with nut allergies.

—

Planted high in the mountainous woods, the tall, coniferous, evergreen Korean pine takes root on solid rocks and stays green through snowstorms, symbolizing our country's natural landscape and the resilient spirit and character of the people.

Despite many wars, foreign invasions, and colonization, we have maintained our national identity like our national tree, the Korean pine, adapting to our natural and changing environment for thousands of years and enduring the struggles of famine, poverty, and abuse. The Korean pine is a sacred companion for us from birth to death, protecting us from evil forces.

The leaves are scaly and deciduous as well as long, like needles, to keep out evil spirits with its sharp needles. We lived in homes that were built mostly with pinewood. On Seolla (설날), the first day of the first lunar month, a pine branch is hung by the gate of a home. It is a symbol that the house guardian god Seongju is keeping out unclean forces. Seongju is the highest deity in the house, overseeing every inch of the house from the shingles of the roof to the safety of the family.

The branches are twisted or knotted and need careful pruning as they grow, much in the way babies need consistent care from their parents. When a baby is born, braided rice grass is hung over the gate for twenty-one days with pine branches and charcoal for protection.

As the tree matures, male cones produce long, slim clusters and the female cones are conical, spreading pollen by the wind, similar to how we reproduce through our encounter with another. As the pine trees age throughout the years, the bark turns tough, like deep wrinkles on our skin, along furrows turning over the earth.

recipe follows

PINE NUT PORRIDGE

잣죽 [jatjuk]

SERVES 4

½ cup (98 g) white or
   (95 g) brown rice
½ cup (68 g) pine nuts
1 tablespoon (15 g)
   packed brown sugar or
   coconut sugar
3 cups (700 ml) filtered
   water
Pinch of salt

The sweet and soothing taste of pine nut porridge is my comfort food whenever I am reminded of my childhood illness. Grandma blessed the porridge by sprinkling pine nuts and told me that this porridge was served to kings to relieve fatigue and fortify their constitution. It improves blood circulation and emotional health, prevents frequent urination, increases virility, and contains antiaging properties due to antioxidants, including vitamins A, B, C, D, and E. There is a saying that three years of eating pine nut porridge would lead one to become an immortal spirit because of its miraculous, medicinal properties.

1. Wash the rice until the water runs clear and then soak the rice for 5 minutes and drain the water. Wash and drain the pine nuts.

2. Combine the pine nuts, rice, and brown or coconut sugar into a food processor. Continue to process while adding water in intervals. Place the mixture in a medium-sized saucepot over medium heat. Slowly bring the liquid to a boil and stir continuously. Lower the heat and simmer for 5 minutes while stirring.

3. Add a pinch of salt and serve hot.

—

I give thanks to the edible seeds of pine trees for the heart-friendly nutrients you give me.

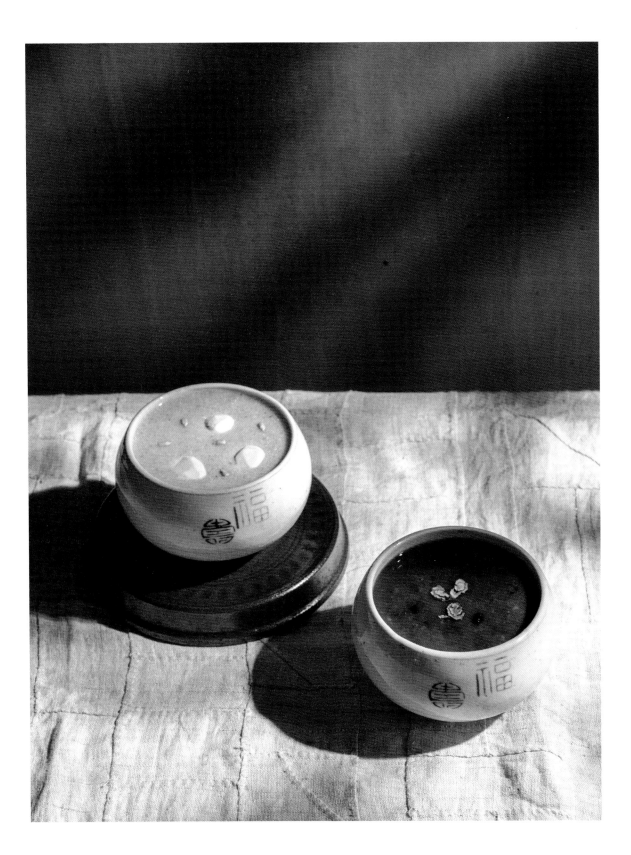

Schisandra 오미자 [omija]

FAMILY: Schisandraceae

GENUS: *Schisandra chinensis*

COMMON NAMES: magnolia berry, five-taste berry

PART USED: fruit

EFFECTIVE QUALITIES: warm, dry, sour, pungent, restoring, raising, stimulating, salty, astringent, stabilizing

NATIVE REGIONS: native to Korea, other parts of Asia

CONSTITUENTS: lignans, phytosterols, organic acids

PROPERTIES: protects liver cells from damaging effects of toxic substances, immunomodulant, promotes regeneration of liver tissue, antioxidant, antimicrobial effects

INDICATED USES: coughs, insomnia, night sweats, physical exhaustion, low sexual drive

NUTRIENTS: vitamins A, C, and E, pectin

—

PREPARATION: Schisandra has numerous medicinal properties that enhances many herbal formulas. Dried schisandra berries are great additions to teas and broths. Power and tincture form is also available.

DOSE: 2–12 grams per day or 2–4 milliliters three times per day

CAUTION: While side effects with schisandra are rare, they may include an upset stomach, decreased appetite, and skin rash. It should not be used during pregnancy.

—

The berries of this deciduous twining shrub are known internationally for giving five flavors—sweetness, sourness, bitterness, saltiness, and pungency. It is found in cool climates throughout woody, montane temperatures in Korea. The berries provide restorative effects on our brain and central nervous system. It tonifies Qi, blood, and essence; it relieves fatigue; and it is an adaptogen that helps respond to unproductive stress. This medicinal berry also protects liver cells from damaging effects of toxic substances and promotes regeneration of liver tissue.

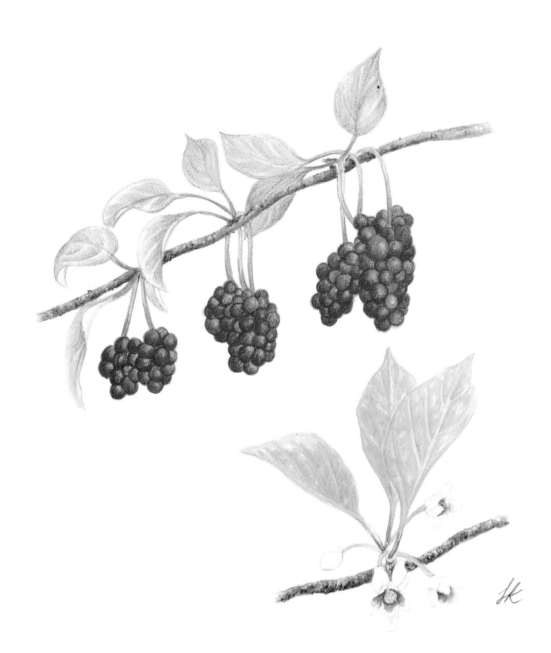

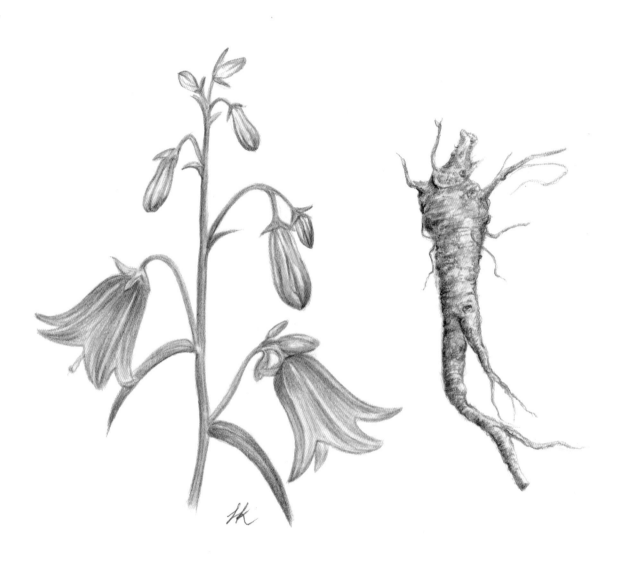

Three Leaf Ladybell
잔대 [jandae]

FAMILY: Campanulaceae

GENUS: *Adenophora triphylla*

COMMON NAMES: ladybell, Japanese ladybell

PART USED: root

EFFECTIVE QUALITIES: antifungal, expectorant, cardiotonic, lung protective

NATIVE REGIONS: Korea, China, Japan

CONSTITUENTS: saponins, triterpenes

PROPERTIES: antifungal, expectorant, cardiotonic

INDICATED USES: cough, bronchial catarrh, sputum

NUTRIENTS: minerals, amino acids, fatty acids, vitamins E and C

—

PREPARATION: Three leaf ladybell root is usually boiled and eaten in soups.

DOSE: 10–15 grams dried in decoction; 15–60 grams fresh in decoction

CAUTION: Three leaf ladybell should not be used during pregnancy.

—

Grown in grassy lowlands and mountains, the elegant ladybell blooms bell-shaped pale blue flowers in the late summer or early fall with seeds ripening in late fall. Once the roots are harvested, the outer layer is stripped off and sun-dried for medicinal use. The roots have a light sweet taste and slight bitterness. There are at least ten species of Adenophora ladybells, the most common being purple ladybells.

Motherwort 익모초 [ikmocho]

FAMILY: Lamiaceae

GENUS: *Leonurus cardiaca*

COMMON NAMES: throw-wort, Lion's tail

PARTS USED: flower, leaves

EFFECTIVE QUALITIES: cool, dry, vital stimulant, relaxant, diffusive, bitter, pungent, astringent, relaxing, calming, stimulating, restoring

NATIVE REGIONS: Asia, Europe

CONSTITUENTS: essential oil, alkaloids, choline, trace minerals, malic acids

PROPERTIES: cardiorelaxant, nervine tonic, sedative, hypnotic, emmenogogue, antispasmodic, antihypertensive, astringent

INDICATED USES: slows an elevated rate of heartbeat, relieves problems with nervous disorders and menstruation

NUTRIENTS: calcium, potassium chloride

—

PREPARATION: Internally, motherwort is used as an infusion or tincture. External preparations are used as suppositories for vaginal infections and poultices for tissue.

DOSE: Infusion: 8–14 grams; tincture: 2–5 milliliters at 1:3 strength in 45 percent ethanol

CAUTION: As a uterine stimulant, motherwort should not be used during pregnancy. Handling it may cause skin irritation to sensitive individuals.

—

We call upon motherwort on Dano Day (단오), the fifth day of the fifth lunar month, as a totem during strong yang energy. We worship the sky deity during the end of sowing season on Dano Day and perform ritualistic ceremonies with herbs such as hair cleaning with Korean iris extract to repel evil forces. Motherwort was used to ward off evil spirits and bad luck from the family. Pregnant women in particular would carry a sachet of motherwort to protect their unborn child. A motherwort decoction is used routinely after birth to help the uterus contract, reducing pain and stopping bleeding.

Motherwort has a deep connection to the uterus and heart, and the energetic connection between both organs helps release tension caused by emotional and mental stress. For women, it is used to promote milk flow and relieve menopausal symptoms and menstrual pains. It is used as a remedy for delayed menstrual periods, flatulence, and hyperthyroidism.

Its medicinal properties have been used in Eastern medicine as a relaxing agent to treat anxiety, insomnia, heart palpitations, and uterine contractions. Motherwort can also be applied to the skin to relieve itching and shingles.

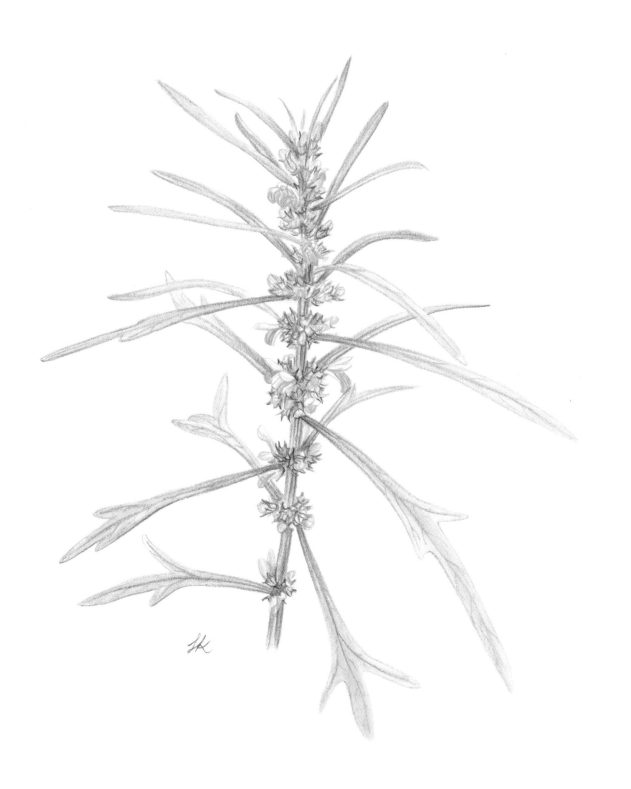

Poria Mushroom
백복령 [baekbokryeong]

FAMILY: Polyporaceae

GENUS: *Wolfiporia extensa*

COMMON NAME: Poria cocos

PART USED: filaments under cap

EFFECTIVE QUALITIES: mild, neutral, somewhat sweet

NATIVE REGIONS: East Asia, Southeast Asia

CONSTITUENTS: polysaccharides, triterpenoids, histidine

PROPERTIES: demulcent, digestive, anti-inflammatory, tonic, diuretic, sedative, antitumor, antioxidant, immunomodulatory, antiaging, anti-hepatitis, anti-diabetes, anti-hemorrhagic fever

INDICATED USES: psoriasis, contact dermatitis, digestive problems, anxiety, insomnia, diabetes, strengthens immune system

NUTRIENTS: fatty acids, sterols, choline, steroids, potassium salts, amino acids, enzymes

—

PREPARATION: Poria usually comes in powdered form and is taken with boiled water as a decoction.

DOSE: Decoction: 9–15 grams per day

CAUTION: There are no known side effects associated with long-term poria use. People taking antidiuretic medications should avoid taking poria as it promotes diuresis.

—

Poria mushroom filaments have been used in Eastern medicine for more than two thousand years to treat physical and mental conditions such as anxiety, fatigue, tension, fluid retention, insomnia, and digestive issues. It is associated with the heart, pancreas, lung, and kidney in Eastern medicine. There are studies showing that poria has treated people with diabetes, Alzheimer's disease, and cancer due to the bioactive components such as triterpenoids, fatty acids, sterols, enzymes, and polysaccharides.

recipe follows

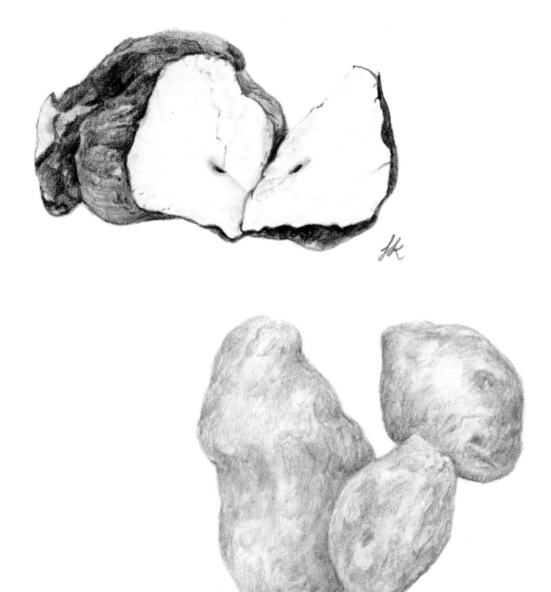

MUSHROOM MEDLEY SOUP

버섯 수프 [beoseot supeu]

½ bundle enoki
  mushrooms
10 shiitake mushrooms
¼ pound (115 g) shimeji
  mushrooms
3 teaspoons sesame oil
½ teaspoon chopped
  garlic
½ cup (120 ml) beef or
  vegetable broth
3 cups (700 ml) water
1 teaspoon poria
  mushroom powder
1 scallion, sliced
Salt and pepper, to taste
Cooked rice, for serving

Often forged in the woods, bioactive compounds of mushrooms are used for medicine and meals. The medley of mushrooms in this soup gives us rich protein and fiber to protect and mitigate the risk of developing serious diseases like Alzheimer's, heart disease, and diabetes. The pine mushroom is one of the most treasured edible mushrooms and is often called the truffle of Asia.

1. Wipe the mushrooms with a damp cloth to clean. Remove the shiitake mushroom stems and slice the caps into thin pieces. In a stockpot, warm the sesame oil over low heat. Add the garlic and broth and cook for 2 to 3 minutes. Add the water, raise the heat, and bring to a boil.

2. Remove any impurities that come to the surface of the water. Add the mushrooms and poria mushroom powder and simmer for 5 minutes. Add the scallions and season with salt and pepper. Serve hot with a bowl of rice.

—

A kingdom of their own, a network of roots connecting trees and plants creating symbiotic relationships.

Ginkgo 은행 [eunhaeng]

FAMILY: Ginkgoaceae

GENUS: *Ginkgo biloba*

COMMON NAMES: ginkgo biloba, maidenhair tree

PARTS USED: nuts, leaves

EFFECTIVE QUALITIES: astringent, neutral, dry, tonic, restoring, decongesting, relaxing, raising, diluting

NATIVE REGION: Asia (now cultivated worldwide)

CONSTITUENTS: terpene lactones, flavone glycosides

PROPERTIES: stimulates blood circulation, decongestant, restorative, protective from free-radical damage

INDICATED USES: vitalizes heart and blood, restores brain and nerves, reduces free radicals, strengthens veins and capillaries

NUTRIENTS: vitamins A and C, niacin, sodium, phosphorus, copper, niacin

—

PREPARATION: Tincture, fluid extracts, or capsule form

DOSE: 120 milligrams daily, in two or three divided doses of 50:1 extract

CAUTION: Ginkgo biloba is very safe; however, there have been isolated cases of gastrointestinal disorders and dizziness in patients taking excess amounts, so please take in moderation.

—

Ginkgo biloba is the oldest living fossil tree in the world. As the seasons transition into fall, the green fan-shaped leaves turn yellow, and as the leaves spin and spiral down to the ground covering sidewalks, I'm reminded of the yellow brick road from *The Wizard of Oz*. Each step on the yellow ginkgo road is an action to explore with others on our life journey, finding our way home.

Ginkgo is mainly cultivated for its nuts and leaves. The most important constituents are dried leaf extracts that have many cognitive benefits such as boosting memory and concentration. Flavone glycosides and terpene lactones in ginkgo provide blood flow to protect brain tissue from the damaging effects of free radicals and toxins. There have been various clinical trials that found ginkgo to be effective in treating patients with dementia. The bioactive chemicals in ginkgo have beneficial medicinal properties that promote health and fight diseases such as dementia, cancer, obesity, and diabetes. Ginkgo has been used as food and medicine for centuries and serves as a natural remedy for treating a wide range of symptoms.

Korean Perilla 깻잎 [kkaenip]

FAMILY: Lamiaceae

GENUS: *Perilla frutescens*

COMMON NAMES: perilla mint, beefsteak plant, purple perilla, shiso, wild coleus, blueweed, Joseph's coat, rattlesnake weed

PARTS USED: leaves, seeds

EFFECTIVE QUALITIES: fragrant, grassy, slightly acerbic, minty licorice

NATIVE REGION: East Asia

CONSTITUENTS: phytochemicals, hydrocarbons, alcohols, aldehydes, furans, ketones, perillaldehyde, limonene, linalool, beta-caryophyllene, menthol

PROPERTIES: anti-inflammatory, antibacterial, expectorant, carminative, emollient, diaphoretic

INDICATED USES: seasonal allergies, asthma, nausea, muscle spasms, sunstroke

NUTRIENTS: quercetin, potassium, rosmarinic acid, luteolin, chrysoeriol, catechin, caffeic acid, ferulic acid, essential oils

—

PREPARATION: Perilla is prepared in culinary forms or as a decoction.

DOSE: Decoction: 3–12 grams

CAUTION: There are no known side effects from taking large doses of perilla leaf, nor are there any known drug interactions, but if you are pregnant or have a preexisting medical condition, please consult with your Eastern medical practitioner or healthcare provider.

—

I will always remember the aroma of perilla leaves as it was the scent of Grandma, earth and minty. Every year, perilla leaves flourished in her garden, and there were endless rows of perilla leaves for anyone to harvest. She was always so generous with others and gave the fruits of her labor to everyone.

Perilla is an herb whose leaves and seeds are used to make culinary dishes and herbal medicine. The leaves and seeds have been used to treat asthma, nausea, and sunstroke; to induce sweating; and to reduce muscle spasm. The phytochemical compounds and flavonoids in perilla leaves have been shown to help fight depression, diabetes, asthma, and cancer. Perilla plants are very easy to grow in your garden and are a great foraging snack. The raw leaves have a very earthy and cuminlike flavor to them. Korean seasoning on the leaves enhances the flavor, and you can just eat the seasoned leaves and rice alone.

PICKLED PERILLA LEAVES

깻잎 장아찌 [kkaetip jangajji]

SERVES 4

30 large perilla leaves
10 tablespoons (150 ml)
 soy sauce
1 teaspoon Korean chile
 flakes
1 teaspoon minced garlic
2 tablespoons (40 g)
 honey or (30 g) brown
 sugar
2 tablespoons (12 g)
 finely chopped scallions
Cooked rice, for serving

Similar to layering tomato sauce on lasagna noodles, perilla leaves are marinated with a soy seasoning in which you layer the sauce between each perilla leaf. This side dish in Korean cuisine is known as pickled perilla leaves. Once the leaves are marinated in the soy seasoning for at least 12 hours, it is ready to be eaten. Perilla leaves can also be used as a wrap like lettuce wraps.

1. Wash the perilla leaves. In a medium bowl, whisk together the soy sauce, chile flakes, garlic, honey or brown sugar, and scallions. Layer each perilla leaf with a spoonful of the seasoned soy sauce like lasagna. Enjoy the pickled perilla leaves with a bed of rice!

—

As time goes by, the simple truth about plants is that they are here to teach us the lessons of life.

FRUIT AND PERILLA SUMMERS

Texas sun beating down our backs as we harvest perilla leaves, Korean pears, and melons—

My heart beats when my sister sings her melodies as she peels the skin off a Korean pear.

Carefully cutting a plate full of fruit, she presents it to the family, as the perfect cut fruit is a reflection of her skills and potential for a fortunate marriage.

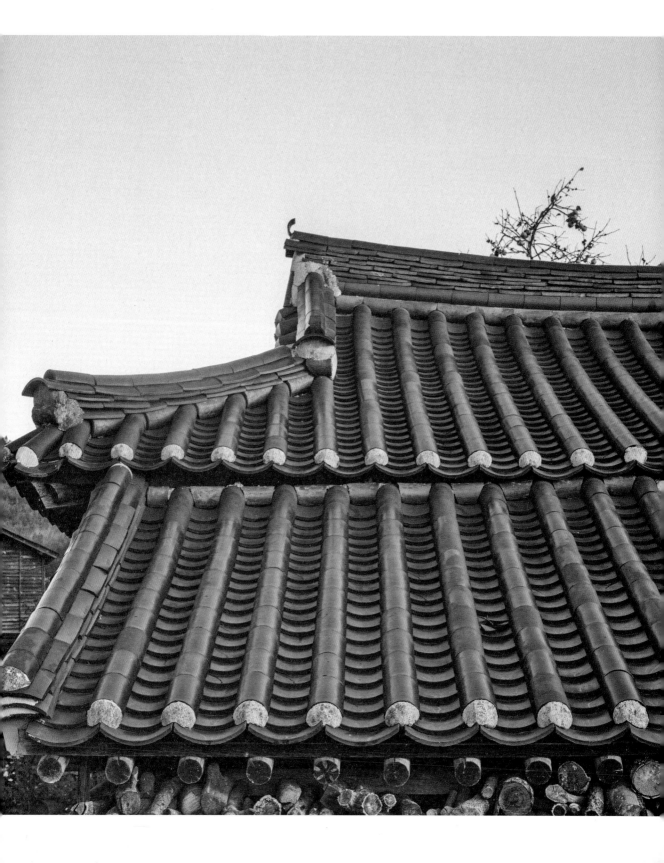

7 MOON HERBS OF WINTER

☷ 감 [gam]

MOON SONG

Mr. Moon told me to pick a direction—North, South, East, or West.
He spun me around three times and pointed to the moon.
Looking straight into my almond eyes he said, "You can do whatever you want to do."

Mrs. Song came along and turned on a light and airy melody so our frenetic thoughts would
tune off. Listen to the Moon Song—it's inside you.

You can do anything you want to.
It's your Moon Song.

We have a divine sense of being when we look into the moon.
And moon songs come true only if we start to call for hands from above.

So listen to the Moon Song.
It's deep inside you.

THE WINTER SOLSTICE

Dongji (동지), the winter solstice, is the shortest day of the year, in terms of sunlight, but it is no less significant, and it is often referred to as the Little New Year. Within the "cup is half full" optimism is the understanding that though the winter solstice gives us the least amount of sunlight, it is also the start of our days growing brighter and brighter. Like nearly all other cultures around the world, Korean culture connects its seasonal holidays with food. Winter solstice is traditionally celebrated by eating red bean porridge (patjuk, 팥죽), a tradition derived from the belief that consuming red beans emits positive Qi and wards off evil spirits.

RED BEAN PORRIDGE

팥죽 [patjuk]

SERVES 4

½ cup (90 g) dried red beans
½ cup (98 g) white or (95 g) brown rice
4 cups (946 ml) water
1 to 2 teaspoons salt

Red beans have warming properties, and they are a great remedy for various liver conditions as well as for treating pneumonia, colds, and flus. Red beans stimulate digestion and are diuretic, so those who are underweight and frequently urinate should avoid consuming large amounts of red beans.

The consistency of porridges varies when the ratio of water to rice changes. The ideal ratio is 3 cups (700 ml) of water to 1 cup (195 g) of rice. Temperature is important to monitor when making porridge, or juk. Cook the ingredients at medium heat until the porridge comes to a boil and then decrease the heat and simmer.

1. In separate bowls, wash and soak the red beans and rice. In a pan, bring the red beans to a boil over medium heat. Reduce the heat to simmer and cook until soft. Drain the beans, reserving the liquid in a separate bowl.

2. In a stockpot, bring the rice and red bean liquid to a boil over medium-high heat. Reduce the heat to simmer and cook until the rice is soft. When the rice is ready, add the red beans. Stir and simmer for 5 minutes. Serve the porridge seasoned with salt.

—

We are comforted by the warmth of red beans and rice, simple yet hearty.

WINTER CLOUD

Morning by morning
Day by day
Our days go round and round
Lost and found.
I think of you over and over again.

Dear brother,
I wanted you to stay.
Stay a little longer, so I can see the love and laughter in
your eyes.
Now you're a cloud looking down at me—free and resting
in peace.

Free
        and
                resting in peace.

To my brother—you never got to take a breath of air on this earth, and I never truly met you, but you still exist as an element of the family, a piece of our history. Umma (mother, 엄마) said she saw my brother in her dream. He was standing at the edge of a waterfall, waving until the beat of pansori made his heart stop. Pansori, traditional Korean songs that pass on rituals from generation to generation, isn't just about singing a song. The voice may represent the wind, trees, waterfalls, or everyday people. It also represents different emotions of sadness or anger.

When we listen to pansori closely, we can feel the stories of love, death, tradition, or honor through the emotions conveyed by sound and breath. When we stand near a waterfall, the scenery is breathtaking. And if we listen closely, the sounds of waterfalls are all different based on their size: Large waterfalls create a loud thunderous sound, whereas small waterfalls create a calmer fluid sound. My waterfall roars as I cascade along the landscapes of my life. My brother shares so many significant silences and contemplative moments with me—a sister/brother bond.

Next time you come across a waterfall, stand near it and sing a song that connects you to Mother Nature. Even if you do not like the sound of your voice, just try to sing along with the waterfall   you may surprise yourself.

The flowing streams of the Han River, a well of living water, feeds herbs that need moisture. It is important to note that one significance of the Han River is the miracle for which it is referred. In the years following Korea's independence in 1945, the country suffered through military occupation and the horrific cost of the Korean War. Through the policies and efforts of President Park Chung Hee, Korea saw a swift renaissance that resulted in robust growth in its infrastructure, manufacturing hub, military, trade, and overall prosperity that is called "the Miracle on the Han River."

WINGS TO FLY

Appa (Papa) always said to fly high like a bird and
follow the Moon.

When you soar far and wide, always remember to help
birds with broken wings.

Appa used to say that the swallow is a bird with a rich mythology and a friend to humankind. Ornithologically, swallows are valued for the way they rid man of unwanted insects and inspire the creatives, poets, and engineers alike with their movements and song. Among the writers affected by this swift bird are Aristotle, Shakespeare, T.S. Eliot, Oscar Wilde, and Aesop. In ancient Greece, the swallow was associated with Aphrodite, the goddess of love, and was seen as an emissary of good luck and happiness.

One story Appa used to share was the Korean folktale of two brothers, Heungbu and Nolbu. Once upon a time, there were two brothers. The oldest, Nolbu, was known to be selfish and greedy, and soon after their father died, he kicked out his younger brother, Heungbu, and his family. With no place to go, Heungbu lived poorly and struggled to feed his family. One day, Heungbu spotted an injured swallow and fixed its broken leg, enabling it to fly again. The following spring, the swallow came back to thank Heungbu for his kindness and gave him a pumpkin seed to express gratitude. Heungbu planted it in the soil, and it grew into a large pumpkin. Once Heungbu cut the pumpkin in half, money and jewels poured out of the pumpkin.

His greedy brother, Nolbu, heard about Heungbu's fortune and decided to reenact his brother's luck by purposely breaking a swallow's leg and fixing it to receive a seed. Soon after, the swallow came back with a seed, and Nolbu immediately planted it, anticipating treasures like his brother's pumpkin. Once Nolbu harvested and cut the pumpkin in half, thieves popped out and stole all his property, leaving him homeless and in poverty. Nolbu went to his rich younger brother and begged for forgiveness. His kind-hearted brother forgave Nolbu for his selfish acts and took him in, and they lived happily and peacefully. The moral of this folklore is about living with integrity and being content with what is given to us.

> Eyes on the skies
> Our wings are wide
> Feelings so confound
> > We pray for justice
> > We pray for courage
> > We pray for peace
> We will fly with open wings, far and wide

Sweet Wormwood
개똥 쑥 [gaettong ssuk]

FAMILY: Compositae

GENUS: *Artemisia annua*

COMMON NAMES: sweet annie, wormwood

PART USED: herb

EFFECTIVE QUALITIES: aromatic, somewhat astringent, moist, decongesting, restoring

NATIVE REGIONS: Korea, China, Japan, Siberia to Eastern Europe

CONSTITUENTS: bitter principles, volatile oil

PROPERTIES: plasmodicidal, anti-inflammatory

INDICATED USES: stimulates immunity and clears toxic heat, reduces fever and inflammation, stimulates the brain and nerves

NUTRIENTS: essential oils, flavonoids, artemisinin

—

PREPARATION: tea extract, powder, capsule forms

DOSE: 3 grams of powdered sweet wormwood per day

CAUTION: Wormwood should not be used during pregnancy. If you have any chronic health issues or take medications, please consult with your Eastern medical practitioner or healthcare provider before using wormwood.

—

Sweet wormwood has been used for centuries in Asia to treat fever and diseases. Many infectious microbial and viral diseases have been shown to respond to sweet wormwood, and many countries around the world use the plant as a medicinal tea.

Native to temperate Asia, sweet wormwood produces an extract that's used in traditional medicine to fight malaria. Named after Artemis, the Greek goddess of hunting and childbirth, the herb is rather bitter (as in "bitter as wormwood"). It is actually a strong insecticide and even has properties toxic to cancer cells. There have been recent studies that the extracts from the leaves of sweet wormwood can inhibit the COVID virus.

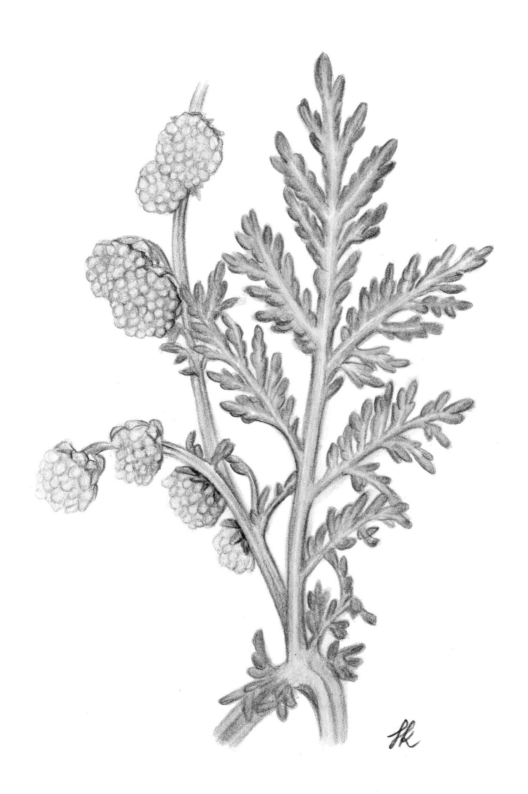

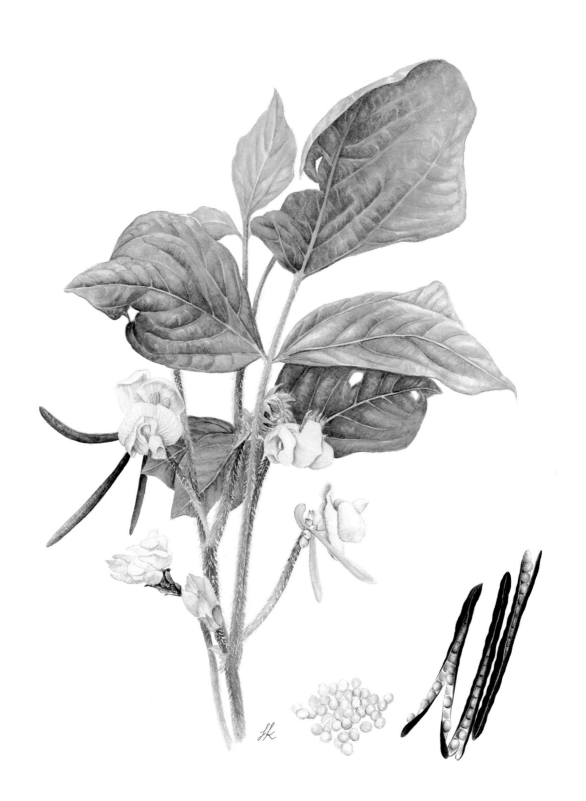

Mung Bean 녹두 [nokdu]

FAMILY: Fabaceae

GENUS: *Vigna radiata*

COMMON NAMES: green gram, monggo

PART USED: seeds

EFFECTIVE QUALITIES: slightly sweet, nutty, crisp, clean

NATIVE REGION: South Asia

CONSTITUENTS: polyphenolics

PROPERTIES: antioxidant, high in fiber, antifungal, antimicrobial, folate-rich

INDICATED USES: lowers cholesterol, lowers blood pressure, aids digestive health, lowers blood sugar levels

NUTRIENTS: vitamin C, iron, calcium, magnesium

—

PREPARATION: Mung beans are primarily used in culinary dishes such as fermented mung bean paste.

DOSE: 1 cup (207 g) of dried mung beans

CAUTION: No adverse effects have been reported in patients taking mung bean.

—

Mung beans were an essential legume when Korea was struck by famine during the Joseon dynasty. Korean mung bean pancakes, bindaetteok, were known as commoner's food as they were served to vagabonds to stave off hunger. Now, everyone loves bindaetteok, and it is a staple Korean cuisine.

The mung bean originated in India around 1500 BCE. It is versatile and popular in dishes across multiple continents. It can be used to feed livestock and as a substitute for meat because of its high protein content. It is also used as a fertilizer for future crops. Fermented mung beans contain live enzymes and bacteria that restores the intestinal flora and helps assimilate nutrients in the digestion process.

recipe follows

MUNG BEAN PANCAKES

빈대떡 [bindaetteok]

Mung bean pancakes are packed with nutritious and hearty ingredients, and they are usually served as a shared appetizer. This mung bean pancake is gluten-free and super easy to make.

MAKES 2 LARGE PANCAKES OR 4 SMALL PANCAKES

1 cup (207 g) dried mung beans
1 cup (110 g) cauliflower rice
¾ cup (175 ml) water
1 cup (85 g) soybean sprouts
1 cup (100 g) kimchi
4 scallions, sliced
1 medium carrot, sliced
2 cloves garlic, minced
1 chile pepper
1 large egg
1 teaspoon sesame oil, plus more for oiling the pan
1 teaspoon black pepper
2 teaspoons kosher salt

1. Soak the mung beans in water for 8 hours or overnight.

2. Drain the mung beans. In a food processor, combine the mung beans, cauliflower rice, and water until creamy. Transfer the mixture to a large bowl. Add the soybean sprouts, kimchi, scallions, carrot, and garlic. Stir to combine. Stir in the chile pepper, egg, sesame oil, pepper, and salt to the bowl.

3. Heat a large skillet over medium-high heat. Add 1 to 2 tablespoons (15 to 28 ml) of sesame oil. Add about 1 cup (235 ml) of batter and spread with a spoon to make a 6-inch (15 cm) pancake. Cook for 2 to 3 minutes until the bottom turns light golden brown.

4. Flip it and cook until the second side turns golden brown. Flip it over once more and cook the first side for another 2 minutes. Add more oil as needed. Set the finished pancake aside on a plate and repeat to cook the remaining batter.

—

We hit mung when we empty our heart and mind to bring more space for peace and creativity.

Soybean 콩 [kong]

FAMILY: Fabaceae

GENUS: *Glycine max*

COMMON NAMES: soja bean, soya bean

PARTS USED: bean, sprout

EFFECTIVE QUALITIES: sweet, nutty, neutral

NATIVE REGION: Asia

CONSTITUENTS: lipids, proteins, carbohydrates, flavonoids, triterpenoid saponins, phytochemicals, phytic acid, isoflavones, saponins, tocopherols

PROPERTIES: cholesterol and triglyceride reducing, liver protective, estrogenlike, antioxidant

INDICATED USES: skin protection, controls weight gain and cholesterol levels, balances hormones, manages diabetes, promotes heart health, treats sleep disorder and depression

NUTRIENTS: vitamins K_1 and B, manganese, phosphorus, folate, copper, thiamine

—

PREPARATION: Soybeans are used in culinary dishes and often fermented as soybean paste for soups and dips.

DOSE: 5–10 grams

CAUTION: Avoid taking large amounts of soy if you have a history of kidney stones. Soybeans are toxic if eaten raw and must be thoroughly cooked before consuming.

—

"Where a soybean is planted, soybean grows and where the red bean is planted, red bean grows" is a Korean proverb. It means that everything in this world has a specific reason, and we should search for the root causes and foundations.

Soybeans contain large amounts of phytic acid, minerals, and vitamins. Soymilk and tofu are made from unfermented soybeans. Soy sauce, soybean paste, natto, and tempeh are made from fermented soybeans.

SOYBEAN SPROUTS SOUP

콩나물국 [kongnamulguk]

SERVES 4

1 cup (85 g) fresh
   soybean sprouts
½ cup (52 g) mung bean
   sprouts
1 teaspoon chopped
   garlic
1 tablespoon (15 ml)
   sesame oil
3 cups (700 ml) water
½ teaspoon anchovy
   powder
Salt and pepper, to taste
2 scallions, sliced
Cooked rice, for serving

Bean sprout soup is good for weight loss, antiaging, liver problems, jaundice, fatigue, and dementia.

1. Trim the roots from the bean sprouts and then wash them thoroughly. In a stockpot, add the bean sprouts, garlic, sesame oil, and water. Cover and bring to a boil over medium-high heat. Reduce the heat to simmer and cook for 10 minutes.

2. Stir in the anchovy powder and season with salt and pepper. Add the scallion and then remove from the heat. Allow the soup to cool. Serve it cold with a bowl of rice.

—

We sing melodies when eating musical note-shaped soybean sprouts!

additional recipes follow

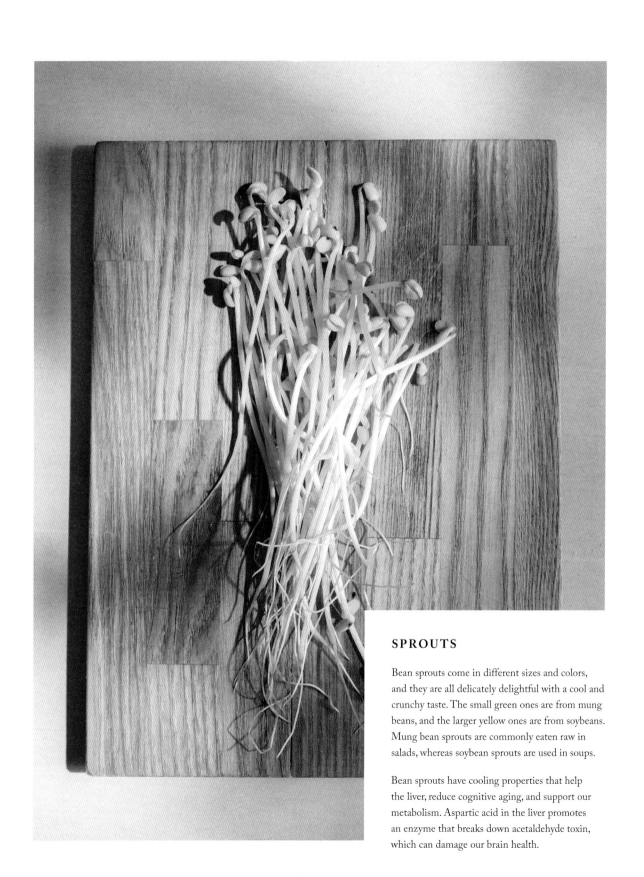

SPROUTS

Bean sprouts come in different sizes and colors, and they are all delicately delightful with a cool and crunchy taste. The small green ones are from mung beans, and the larger yellow ones are from soybeans. Mung bean sprouts are commonly eaten raw in salads, whereas soybean sprouts are used in soups.

Bean sprouts have cooling properties that help the liver, reduce cognitive aging, and support our metabolism. Aspartic acid in the liver promotes an enzyme that breaks down acetaldehyde toxin, which can damage our brain health.

SPROUT SALAD

콩나물 무침 [kongnamul muchim]

SERVES 4

1 pound (455 g) soybean
  sprouts
2 teaspoons sesame oil
2 teaspoons sesame seeds
1 clove garlic, chopped
1 scallion, chopped
Pinch of salt
Cooked rice, for serving

These crunchy and nutritious sprouts help lower cholesterol and help prevent high blood pressure, stroke, and hardening of blood vessels. Soybeans are packed with protein and low in fat. This salad is great for people who have high blood pressure, high cholesterol, and poor blood circulation.

1. Trim the roots from the bean sprouts and then wash them thoroughly. Bring a saucepan of water to a boil over medium heat. Add the sprouts, cover the pan, and bring back to a boil. Boil for 5 to 7 minutes until the sprouts look tender yet crisp, being mindful not to overheat the sprouts. Drain the sprouts and allow them to cool slightly.

2. In a medium bowl, combine the sesame oil, sesame seeds, garlic, scallions, and salt. Add the sprouts and mix thoroughly. Serve as a vegetable side dish with rice.

—

With this light and crisp salad, we enjoy the breezy and crunchy days.

PICKLED SOYBEANS

콩장 [kongjang]

MAKES 1 PINT (473 ML)

1 cup (186 g) soybeans
3 cups (700 ml) rice
  vinegar

Soybeans are known to strengthen the pancreas, which enhances insulin production. They are commonly used to help prevent and treat diabetes by maintaining optimal blood sugar level.

1. Wash and dry the soybeans. Add them to a 32-ounce (946 ml) mason jar and then pour over the vinegar. Cover with a lid and store in a cool, dark place for 1 week.

2. Eat 7 to 10 beans daily and chew thoroughly for good absorption. Store pickled soybeans in the refrigerator.

—

Strengthen your pancreas by picking three words, then eat.

Hope	Grace	Honesty
Longevity	Trust	Abundance
Justice	Peace	Wisdom
Laughter	Gratitude	Forgiveness

THE UNKNOWN KINGDOM

Mushrooms are a mystery to many, and I sometimes wonder if the fungi kingdom will still exist after our mushroom obsession ends. It takes years and decades to grow mushrooms from fallen and decayed trees. How will our ecosystem sustain if we are overharvesting? At least there are laboratories that cultivate fungi, they say, but what about the real ones in the wild? Are they becoming scarce to wild harvest? The medicine mushrooms are poria, reishi, chaga, and ashwagandha to name a few. Their symbiotic relationships with plants help take in additional nutrients and minerals, and in return, the fungi receives part of the sugars that the plants generate from photosynthesis. Life on the planet wouldn't exist without fungi.

Black Hoof Mushroom
상황버섯 [sanghwang buhshut]

FAMILY: Polyporaceae

GENUS: *Phellinus igniarius*

COMMON NAME: fire sponge

PART USED: bracket

EFFECTIVE QUALITIES: woody, earthy

NATIVE REGION: East Asia

CONSTITUENTS: bioactive compounds, polysaccharide, ellagic acid, caffeic acid

PROPERTIES: antiviral, anti-inflammatory, antioxidative, antitumor, immunomodulatory

INDICATED USES: boosts immune system, relieves inflammation, combats certain cancers

NUTRIENTS: flavones, polyphenols

—

PREPARATION: Black hoof mushroom is consumed in tea form, either as a powder or as a dried herb.

DOSE: 1 teaspoon in powder form

CAUTION: If you have any chronic illness or take medications, please consult with your Eastern medical practitioner or healthcare provider before taking black hoof mushrooms.

—

Black hoof mushroom is a member of the Polyporaceae family and is a perennial medicinal and edible fungus that grows on aspen, oak, willow, mulberry, and birch trees. It has a shape similar to a clamshell, and unlike other mushrooms, the black hoof creates new hardy wood layers every year. Similar to our skin, it is constantly renewing its cells so it can regenerate. It is an important medicinal and edible fungus in Asia and has diverse biological activities. In addition to its anticancer benefits, it is great for increasing strength, alleviating hangovers, and treating anemia and menstrual irregularity. In Korea, it is widely consumed as a preventive healthcare product. There have been studies that show pharmacologically active metabolites and polysaccharides help fight cancer cells.

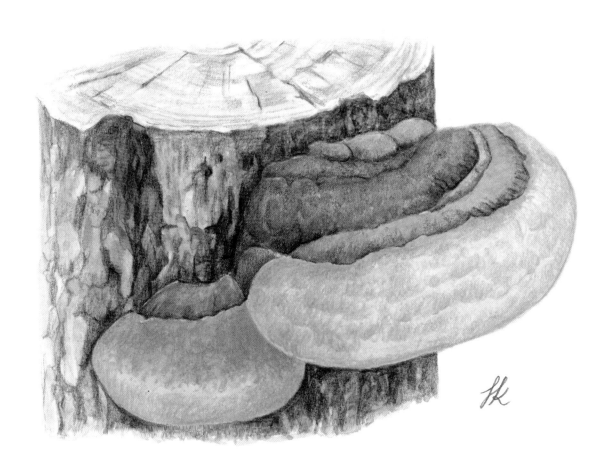

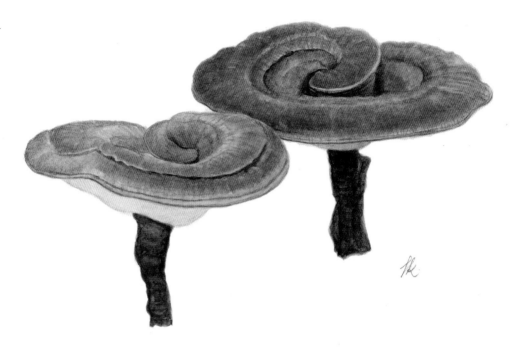

Reishi
영지버섯 [yeonggi buhsuht]

FAMILY: Ganodermataceae

GENUS: *Ganoderma lucidum*

PART USED: entire mushroom

EFFECTIVE QUALITIES: slightly warm, moist, stimulant, nutritive tonic, bitter, neutral, bland, sweet

NATIVE REGION: Asia

CONSTITUENTS: polysaccharides, triterpenes, peptidoglycans

PROPERTIES: immune modulator, antitumor, adrenal restorative, anticarcinogenic, antiallergic, regulates cholesterol, oxygenator, antiaging

INDICATED USES: adaptogen, immune stimulant, immune balancer, allergies, immunodeficiency, cardiac stress, heart palpitations, chronic degenerative disease

NUTRIENTS: calcium, potassium, magnesium, phosphorus, selenium, iron, zinc, copper

—

PREPARATION: Reishi is taken in different forms from powder, tincture, extract, to capsule.

DOSE: Extract: 6–10 grams daily

CAUTION: Reishi may cause dizziness, dry mouth, itching, nausea, and upset stomach. It should not be consumed by individuals taking blood thinners or with low blood pressure. Like with all herbs, consume what you need, and if your body is not adapting well to the herb, then hold off on consuming more.

—

Reishi mushrooms have been used for hundreds of years, mainly in Asia, for the treatment of medical conditions and infections. Currently, it is used in the treatment of cancer and pulmonary disease. Also known as the lingzhi, reishi has been used to improve immune response, improve sleep, and fight fatigue. This is the same mushroom of Korean folklore that brought immortality to Magu, a beautiful woman who lived on Guyu Mountain.

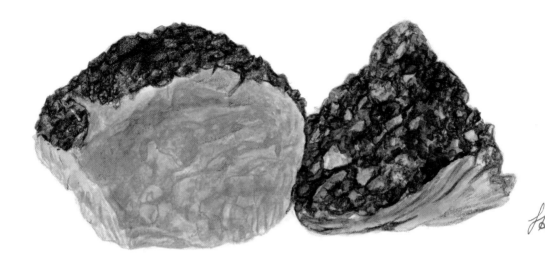

Chaga Mushroom
차가버섯 [chaga buhsuht]

FAMILY: Hymenochaetaceae

GENUS: *Inonotus obliquus*

COMMON NAMES: cinder conk, birch conk, clinker polypore

PART USED: mycelial mass

EFFECTIVE QUALITIES: neutral, mild, earthy, slightly bitter

NATIVE REGION: Asia

CONSTITUENTS: beta-glucans, triterpenoids

PROPERTIES: antitumor, anti-mutagenic, antiviral, anti-diabetic, antioxidant, immunomodulating, anti-inflammatory, pain-relieving effects, boosts energy, increases mental sharpness, reduces fatigue

INDICATED USES: boosts energy, increases mental sharpness, reduces fatigue

NUTRIENTS: vitamins D and B, potassium, fiber, copper, amino acids, rubidium

—

PREPARATION: Chaga is mainly taken in powder form.

DOSE: 2 grams daily

CAUTION: Chaga should not be used during pregnancy or breastfeeding. Some of the compounds may stimulate the immune function, so chaga should be avoided by individuals with autoimmune conditions. Chaga can lower blood sugar, so individuals with diabetes should be careful when using it.

—

Medicinal mushrooms are classified into edible species or extracted species. Extracted species go through an extraction process to make some of the active components bioavailable. Chaga is an extracted species and is native to Korea.

The slow growing process of chaga can take years and even decades to develop on birch trees. Thriving in cold and moist conditions, chaga in tea form is commonly sipped during the winter nights. Chaga has many medicinal properties, and the mushroom boosts energy, increases mental sharpness, and reduces fatigue.

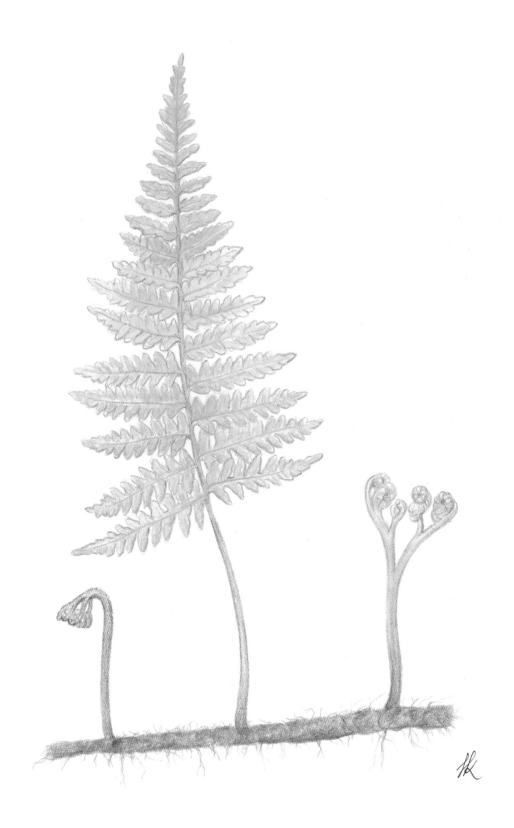

Bracken 고사리 [gosari]

FAMILY: Dennstaedtiaceae

GENUS: *Pteridium aquilinum*

COMMON NAMES: fernbrake, bracken fiddleheads, fiddlehead greens

PARTS USED: stems, fiddleheads

EFFECTIVE QUALITIES: astringent, tonic

NATIVE REGIONS: Eurasia, North America

CONSTITUENTS: flavonoid, phenol, terpenoid compounds

PROPERTIES: diuretic, vermifuge, refrigerant, antiseptic, digestive

INDICATED USES: stomach cramps, headaches, nausea and vomiting, fever, insomnia

NUTRIENTS: vitamins C and B_2, protein, iron, fiber

—

PREPARATION: Bracken fiddleheads are commonly used as a Korean culinary side dish.

DOSE: The young, unfurled shoots are used in culinary preparations, and the roots can be steeped into a tea.

CAUTION: When foraging bracken fiddleheads, please go with someone who is an expert in foraging bracken as parts of the plant are toxic, and it must be prepared properly before consuming.

—

Bracken, also known as gosari in Korean, is a large fern that can grow to be 3 feet (0.9 m) tall.

In Korean culture, the young stem has been eaten for centuries and is praised for its rich amounts of vitamins, antioxidants, and fiber. It is considered "the beef of the mountains" for its high protein content and hearty flavor. The fiddleheads have stems that grow underground, like roots, called rhizomes, which can grow 6 feet (1.8 m) long and can be found in moist areas near riverbanks and meadows.

Bracken root is quite versatile from making baskets to promoting hair growth. It is a common ingredient in soups, fried rice, or mixed steamed in a popular rice dish called bibimbap. There is recent debate concerning the safety of consuming the plant due to the presence of the compound ptaquiloside. After a broad survey of scientific research and literature, blanched and sautéed gosari can be safely consumed. Ptaquiloside is infamous for being volatile at moderate temperatures and degenerates at room temperature. When exposed to boiling temperatures, the carcinogen denatures almost completely.

Deodeok 더덕 [deodeok]

FAMILY: Campanulaceae

GENUS: *Codonopsis lanceolata*

COMMON NAME: lance asiabell

PART USED: root

EFFECTIVE QUALITY: mildly bitter

NATIVE REGIONS: Central Asia, East Asia, South Asia

CONSTITUENTS: phenolic compounds, polyacetylenes, polyphenols, saponins, tannins, triterpene, alkaloids, steroids

PROPERTIES: depurative, anticancer, emmenagogue, galactagogue

INDICATED USES: bronchitis, coughs, spasm, psychoneurosis, cancer, obesity, hyperlipidemia, edema, hepatitis, colitis, amenorrhea, lung injury

NUTRIENTS: calcium

—

PREPARATION: Deodeok root is a common culinary dish and also used as a decoction.

DOSE: Decoction: 9–30 grams

CAUTION: There are no reports of contraindications or side effects when used properly. It should not be taken by individuals with bleeding disorders due to the possibility that it may slow blood clotting.

—

Deodeok is a plant that grows mainly in the mountains and is sometimes referred to as mountain ginseng. Elements found in the deodeok are excellent for absorbing and purging bad cholesterol and fat. In addition, deodeok is good for lung health, reducing inflammation, and regulating sugar for people with diabetes.

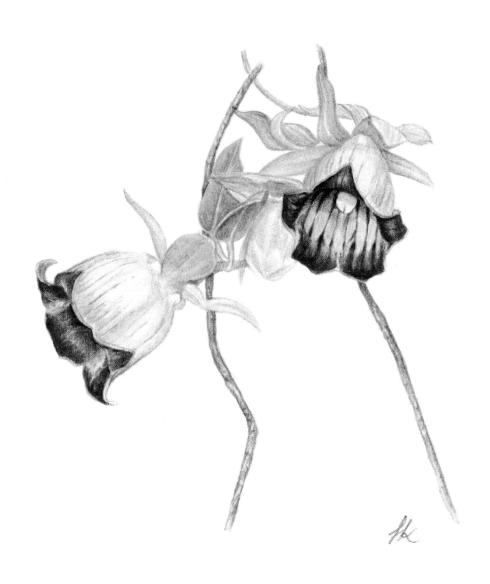
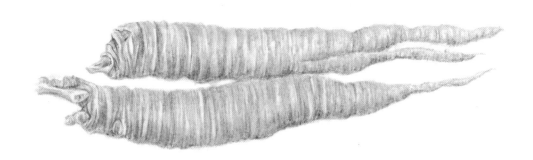

Chestnut 밤 [bam]

FAMILY: Fagaceae

GENUS: *Castanea sativa*

PART USED: fruit

EFFECTIVE QUALITIES: nutty, smoky, hearty

NATIVE REGIONS: Southern Europe, Asia Minor

CONSTITUENTS: tannins, flavonoids, triterpenes, phenolic acids, phytosterols

PROPERTIES: astringent, mild antitussive

INDICATED USES: coughs, bronchitis, minor inflammations of the gastrointestinal tract such as diarrhea

NUTRIENTS: vitamins C and B_6, magnesium, iron, calcium

—

PREPARATION: Chestnuts are a Korean staple and are used in many culinary dishes as well as a healthy snack.

DOSE: 200–400 milligrams by mouth daily for 8 to 12 weeks

CAUTION: There are no reports of contraindications or side effects when used properly.

—

Chestnuts, namely the trees upon which these popular nuts grow, have a rich folklore about one's ability to avoid one's tragic fate. The indigenous tree called nadobamnamu means "I am also a chestnut tree." One day, a Taoist came upon Yi L, son of Duke Yi, whose pen name, Yulgok, translates to "chestnut valley," and who predicted that the boy would one day be eaten by a tiger unless Duke Yi planted a thousand chestnut trees. When his son turned twenty, a menacing stranger demanded the life of the boy. The Duke refused, turning to the thousand chestnut trees he had planted. When he and the stranger counted up the trees, they found that Duke Yi was one tree short. Just then, a nadobamnamu tree stepped forward and proclaimed that he was also a chestnut tree and took the place of the missing tree. At that moment, the stranger turned into a tiger and died, thus fulfilling the Taoist's prophecy. Yulgok avoided this tragic fate and grew up to become a scholar. The folklore's message is that humans can avoid bad fate if they have a chestnut tree nearby and that trees have a rooted mystical connection with people.

Chestnuts and jujubes symbolize fertility and the health of children. The ceremony pyebaek (폐백) is a ritual where the bride is gifted nuts as a wedding pre-ceremony. Then, the bride later visits her in-laws and gives them chestnuts and jujubes as a gift. The in-laws throw them at the bride's skirt for her to catch. However many she catches represents the number of children she will have in the future.

CHESTNUT-GINKGO ENERGY PORRIDGE

밤 은행나무씨죽 [bam eunhaengenergyjuk]

SERVES 4

¼ cup (35 g) dried red beans
20 ginkgo seeds
¼ cup (35 g) raw peanuts
10 chestnuts
½ cup (100 g) short-grain white rice
¼ cup (45 g) sweet rice
5 cups (1.2 L) water
10 dried jujubes
Pine nuts, for garnish

Chestnuts are nutrient-dense, and they increase stamina and energy. The combination of chestnuts, ginkgo, jujubes, and red beans is a traditional remedy that helps lower blood pressure, anemia, and digestive issues. This porridge is great for people who have high blood pressure and experience indigestion.

1. Wash the red beans and soak them overnight.

2. Peel and wash the ginkgo, peanuts, and chestnuts. Place the jujubes in a small bowl, add water to cover, and soak for 30 minutes. Wash the rice and then drain it in a fine-mesh sieve.

3. Add the water, beans, ginkgo, peanuts, chestnuts, white rice, sweet rice, and jujubes to a large stockpot over medium-high heat. Bring to a boil and then reduce the heat and simmer slowly for 7 to 10 minutes. Add water if necessary. When all the ingredients are soft and the liquid is sweet in flavor, remove it from heat. Serve hot, garnished with pine nuts.

—

As I lie under a ginkgo tree, the fan-shaped leaves are waving at me. I breathe in the air and thank Mother Nature for giving me this moment with ginkgo to clear my head and heart.

THE GREAT FULL MOON

On the day of Daeboreum (대보름), the Great Full Moon, we crack nuts with our teeth and celebrate a strong and healthy lunar new year during the first full moon. We climb mountains and brave the cold snow to catch the first rise of the moon as the first person to see the moon rise will have good luck year-round. We cross twelve bridges all night long to strengthen our legs and as steps to good health for all twelve months. We burn the dry grass on ridges between rice fields, and children whirl around cans full of holes with charcoal fire blazing to fertilize the fields and cast away harmful worms that destroy the new crops. We perform these traditions as a remembrance of past generations, for the present, and for a hopeful future.

Ginger 생강 [saeng gang]

FAMILY: Zingiberaceae

GENUS: *Zingiber officinale*

COMMON NAMES: cooking ginger, canton ginger

PART USED: root

EFFECTIVE QUALITIES: hot, pungent, spicy, dry

NATIVE REGIONS: China, India

CONSTITUENTS: volatile oil, pungent, lipids, starch, glycolipids

PROPERTIES: antispasmodic, antacid, anti-inflammatory, analgesic, aromatic, carminative, nervine, stimulant, antiviral, hypoglycemic, circulatory stimulant, expectorant, diaphoretic, sexual tonic

INDICATED USES: morning sickness, motion sickness, indigestion, migraines, cough, respiratory issues, poor circulation, menstrual cramps, fatigue, cold extremities

NUTRIENTS: vitamin C, magnesium

—

PREPARATION: Ginger is commonly used as a culinary herb in raw or powder form. It is also used as tea to aid digestion.

DOSE: 0.5–3 grams

CAUTION: Individuals with gallstones should avoid taking ginger.

—

As a superstar in folk medicine, ginger is a key ingredient in Qi Alchemy's herbal pearls and a great spice to have stocked in your pantry. It adds terrific flavor to our meals, and it is full of medicinal properties. Ginger is loaded with antioxidants. It is used to help relieve an upset stomach, treat the common cold, aid in digestion, and decrease inflammation, making it a popular ingredient in herbal remedies. In recent studies, ginger has also been linked to reducing blood sugar and increasing cognitive function, adding to the versatility of ginger.

The enzymes in ginger support digestion by stimulating bowel movement and reducing intestinal cramping or bloating. One of the main bioactive compounds in ginger is gingerol, which carries powerful antioxidant properties and phytonutrients as it helps prevent inflammation and alleviate pain like arthritis. There also have been studies proving that ginger helps with brain function by improving memory.

recipe follows

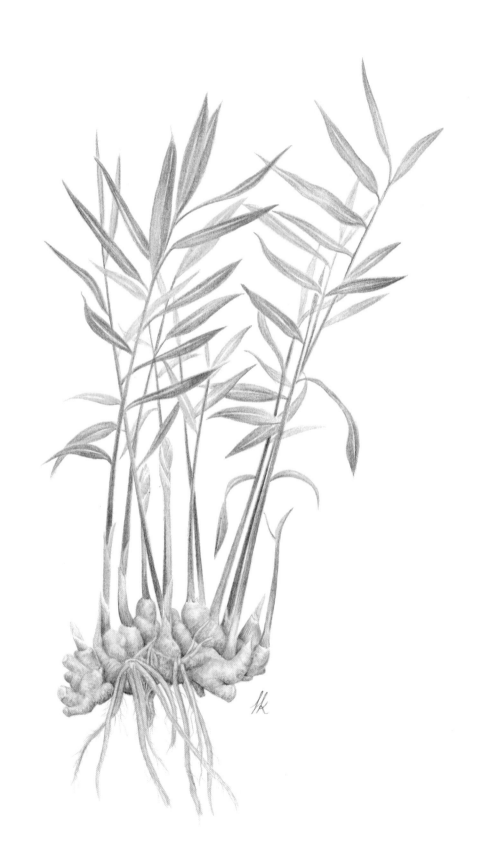

GINGER CINNAMON PUNCH

수정과 [sujeonggwa]

Sujeonggwa is a traditional Korean dessert drink made from ginger and cinnamon and garnished with pine nuts. During the Goryeo dynasty in the 900s, the court ladies would make the drink on New Year's Day by boiling ginger and adding dried persimmons and cinnamon. The ginger aids digestion, and both ginger and cinnamon have antimicrobial properties.

SERVES 4

1 piece (3½ ounces, or 100 g) fresh ginger
2 jujubes
10 cinnamon sticks
8 cups (1.9 L) water

1. Peel the fresh ginger and slice it into thin pieces. Slice the jujubes. Rinse the cinnamon sticks in water. Boil the water over medium-high heat. Add the cinnamon sticks, ginger, and jujubes. Reduce the heat to low and then let it simmer for 20 to 30 minutes.

—

Guide our hearts and protect our gut as we sip on ginger, jujube, and cinnamon.

additional recipes follow

HEART-HEALTHY CINNAMON

Cinnamon is an incredible spice that is part of the Lauraceae family and has been a remedy for many health ailments including heart, cognitive, and respiratory issues. Cinnamon contains antimicrobial and anti-inflammatory properties, helps fight free radicals, and lowers glucose levels in diabetics. Adding cinnamon powder into our morning beverage or breakfast is a simple way to integrate this powerful spice into our lives.

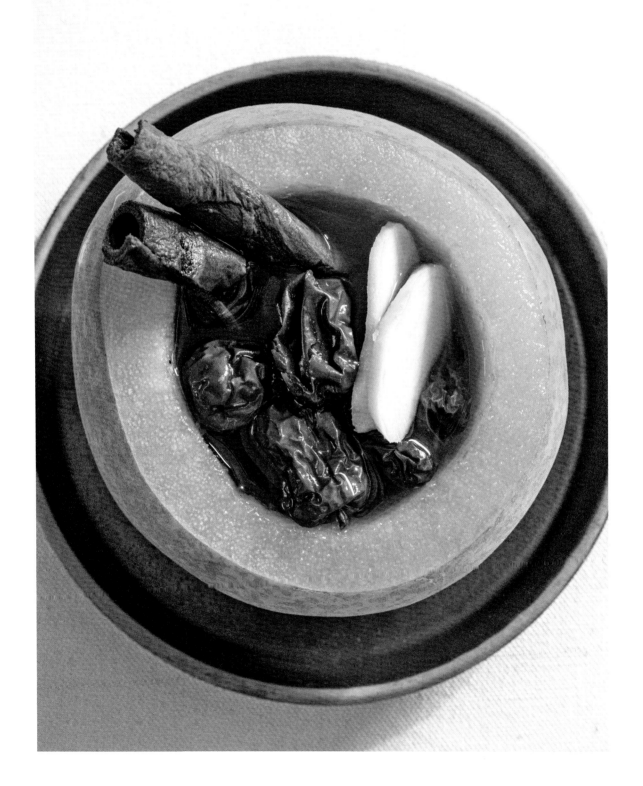

GINGER-TOFU DRESSING (VEGAN)

생강 두부 소스 [saenggang dubu soseu]

MAKES ½ PINT (235 ML)

4 ounces (115 g) silken
   tofu
2 tablespoons (28 ml) rice
   vinegar
2 tablespoons (44 g)
   soybean paste
¼ cup (60 ml) water
2 teaspoons perilla oil
1 clove garlic
1 tablespoon (6 g)
   chopped fresh ginger
1 scallion, chopped

Ginger has a long history in traditional Eastern medicine and is considered a tonic root medicine. It has been used to help digestion, reduce nausea, and help fight the flu and common cold, to name a few. In this creamy vegan dressing, tofu offers a good source of protein and contains all nine essential amino acids. It also contains magnesium, copper, zinc, and vitamin B_1.

1. Add the tofu, vinegar, soybean paste, water, oil, garlic, ginger, and scallion to a blender. Blend until smooth and creamy. Serve immediately or store in an airtight container in the refrigerator for up to 5 days.

—

We ask the universe for smooth transitions as we nourish and pray.

JUICY KOREAN PEAR

한국 배 [hanguk bae]

MAKES 2 PEARS

2 large Korean pears
1 teaspoon sliced ginger
6 tablespoons (120 g)
   honey
Chopped walnuts or
   jujubes, for garnish

Instead of Christmas baskets full of cookies and sweets, Koreans gift pears as they are a delightful and healthy treat. They are often used instead of sugar as a sweetener for marinades, along with soy sauce or vinegar, due to the enzymes that tenderize the meat.

Baked Korean honey pear is a sweet dessert that's free from processed and refined sugar. Pears baked with honey and ginger are medicinal, with cooling properties used to reduce fever and treat colds and sore throats. The dish also contains fiber and vitamins C and K.

1. Preheat the oven to 325°F (170°C, or gas mark 3). Wash the pears and carefully cut off the top of each pear. Using a spoon, remove the core from each pear and gently scoop out a small amount of the flesh to make room. Pour ½ teaspoon of ginger and 3 tablespoons (60 g) of honey inside each pear. Cover each of the pears with its sliced top.

2. Place the pears on a baking sheet and bake for 1 hour or until the fruit softens. Serve warm or cool, garnished with walnuts or jujubes.

—

Taste the sweetness. Open myself fully to give and receive love.

Job's Tears 율무 [yulmu]

FAMILY: Poaceae

GENUS: *Coix lacryma-jobi*

COMMON NAMES: coix seed, adlay millet, Chinese pearl barley

PARTS USED: root, seed

EFFECTIVE QUALITIES: antioxidant effects, antibacterial, antiparasitic

NATIVE REGION: Asia

CONSTITUENTS: coixenolide, phenols, flavonoids, polysaccharides, proteins, fibers, vitamins, oils

PROPERTIES: antimicrobial, antiviral, antitoxin, wound healing, antiaging, diuretic, immunomodulatory, antioxidant, anti-inflammatory

INDICATED USES: arthritis, obesity, hay fever, high cholesterol, cancer, warts, and respiratory tract infections; treats toxoplasmosis

NUTRIENTS: vitamins B_1, B_2, and E, niacin

—

PREPARATION: Decoction or powder are the most common forms.

DOSE: The amount of Job's tears taken depends on the condition being treated; typical decoction: 10–30 grams

CAUTION: Job's tears should not be taken during pregnancy or by individuals with diabetes.

—

Also known as adlay millet or Chinese pearl barley, Job's tears is a tall grain-bearing perennial tropical plant that's part of the grass family. The wild variety of Job's tears has hard-shelled pseudocarps, which are hard, pearly white, oval structures used as beads for making prayer beads. The cultivated type of Job's tears is harvested as a cereal crop and has a soft shell. It is widely used as medicine and tea in Asia. A traditional barley tea called yulmucha (율무차) is made with roasted powdered grains of Job's tears in Korea.

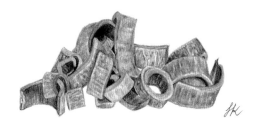

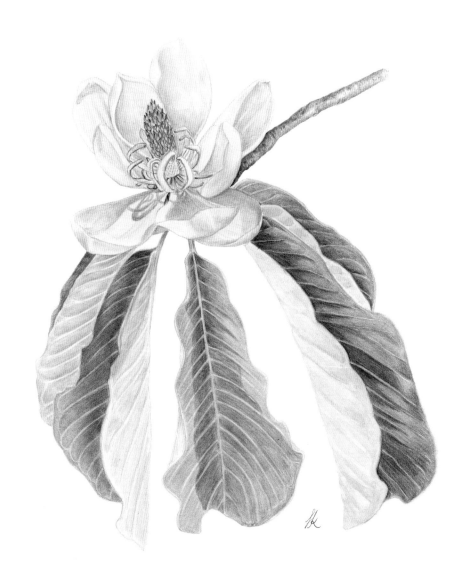

Magnolia Bark 목련 [moklyun]

FAMILY: Magnoliaceae

GENUS: *Magnolia officinalis*

PART USED: bark

EFFECTIVE QUALITIES: bitter, astringent, pungent

NATIVE REGIONS: Korea, Japan

CONSTITUENTS: honokiol, magnolol

PROPERTIES: antihistaminic, analgesic, antihypertensive, uterotonic, antifungal, antibacterial, antiviral

INDICATED USES: headaches, allergic rhinitis, eczema, sleep disorders, improves cortisol levels

NUTRIENTS: vitamin C, carotenoids, tannins, phenols

—

PREPARATION: The bark is harvested first by peeling it from the tree and then dried and boiled until the internal surface of the bark turns a dark red. Then, it is steamed until soft and rolled into cylindrical pieces. The bark is dried again and decocted.

DOSE: Decoction: 3–10 grams

CAUTION: Magnolia bark should not be used during pregnancy.

—

Magnolia bark is an aromatic herb and is an important Eastern medicine ingredient in treating people with sleeping disorders, allergies, and anxiety. The bioactive constituents in magnolia bark, honokiol and magnolol, contain powerful antioxidative properties that help fight against cancer and treat depression.

Korean Sweet Potato
고구마 [goguma]

FAMILY: Convolvulaceae

GENUS: *Ipomoea batatas*

COMMON NAME: sweet potato

PART USED: root vegetable

EFFECTIVE QUALITIES: sweet, dense, fibrous, dry, hearty

NATIVE REGIONS: Polynesia, South America

CONSTITUENTS: phytochemicals, polyphenols, proteins, lipids, carotenoids, anthocyanins, conjugated phenolic acids

PROPERTIES: antioxidant, anti-inflammatory, anti-microbial, antidiabetic, antitumor

INDICATED USES: cardiovascular support, improves brain health and function

NUTRIENTS: vitamins A, B, B_6, and C, manganese, potassium, low-glycemic carbohydrate, dietary fiber

—

PREPARATION: Sweet potatoes are used in many culinary dishes as well as a healthy snack. They are also used in powder form.

DOSE: 4 grams per day

CAUTION: Sweet potatoes have a high oxalate content, which can lead to kidney and gallbladder stones, so consume in moderation.

—

Sweet potatoes are a nutritious root vegetable, and they are considered "medicine of the mountain" in Eastern medicine. They were used for centuries for various medicinal purposes including treating menopause, women's health issues, and coughs. Sweet potatoes boost the immune system and increase overall energy.

Massive famines struck Korea in the late 1600s, leaving people starving, and sweet potato was a hero superfood that saved the population from famine. A farmer introduced and shared his sweet potato seeds to help stop the famine in Busan because the vegetable is resilient in any climate and soil conditions. The first village to grow sweet potatoes in Korea is called Sweet Potato Village. Packed with vitamins, minerals, and fiber, the hearty superfood is a delightful snack or dessert that Koreans love to eat.

SWEET POTATO–MUSHROOM TEA

고구마 버섯차 [goguma-beoseos cha]

MAKES 1 CUP (235 ML)

1 shiitake mushroom
1 cup (235 ml) filtered
 water
1 tablespoon (13 g) sweet
 potato powder
Honey, to taste

Shiitake mushrooms contain twice as much protein as the familiar button mushroom, and according to Eastern medicine, they have many healing properties, including strengthening bones and joints and increasing bone density. The combination of an umami flavor from the shiitake mushroom and a slight sweet flavor brings a third taste that creates a nice flavorful balance to the tea.

1. Wipe the mushroom with a damp cloth to clean. Remove the stem and slice the cap into thin pieces. Boil the water, add the sliced mushroom, reduce the heat to low, and cook for 3 minutes.

2. Place the sweet potato power in a teacup. Pour the water with mushroom slices into the teacup and mix well with a teaspoon. Enjoy this tea hot and add honey to taste.

—

Constant motions of yin and yang, we sip on shiitake mushroom and sweet potato to give us Qi.

Licorice 감초 [gamcho]

FAMILY: Fabaceae

GENUS: *Glycyrrhiza glabra*

COMMON NAMES: licorice root, kanzo, gan cao

PART USED: root

EFFECTIVE QUALITIES: very sweet, neutral in temperature or slightly warm, moistening, strong vital stimulant, relaxant, chi tonic in higher doses, calming, softening

NATIVE REGIONS: Asia, Europe, Middle East

CONSTITUENTS: triterpenoid saponin, flavonoids, oleanane triterpenes, chalcones, polysaccharides, choline, essential oil, bitters, amino acids

PROPERTIES: anti-inflammatory, antiulcer (helps prevent further damage in healing peptic ulcers), antispasmodic, expectorant, demulcent, liver protective, antibacterial, antiviral, antifungal

INDICATED USES: inflammations of upper respiratory tract (such as bronchitis, laryngitis), inflammations of gastrointestinal tract, fatigue, atopic eczema

NUTRIENTS: vitamins A, C, and E

—

PREPARATION: Licorice root is prepared in tea, powder, tincture, or decoction. For greater intestinal absorption, sliced licorice root should be toasted firm before decocting.

DOSE: Decoction: 4–10 grams; tincture: 1–3 milliliters at 1:2 strength in 25 percent ethanol

CAUTION: Licorice root should be avoided in adrenal hyperfunctioning conditions such as hypertension, water retention, hyperglycemia, osteoporosis, and excess secretions or taking certain medications. Seaweed may counteract the properties of licorice root; therefore, seaweed and licorice root should not be taken together.

—

Licorice is widely used as a flavor ingredient in food and herbal medicine, and it is one of those herbs where Eastern and Western herbal medicine intersect. A prominent bioactive compound, glycyrrhizic acid is a natural sweetener with anti-inflammatory properties. Eastern medicine emphasizes treating the Qi deficiency of the pancreas (digestive restorative). Western practice sees its tonic action on the adrenal cortex, pancreas, and gonads (a selective endocrine restorative). In both cases, licorice supports people with fatigue between meals, a loss of appetite, and sweet cravings. Conditions such as hypoglycemia and estrogen deficiency are also treated with licorice.

For centuries, licorice root has been effective in treating stomach ulcers, heartburn, indigestion, and bronchitis. It is used to support the immune system and adrenals. Both Eastern and Western medicine have made use of licorice's anti-infective, anti-inflammatory, and antiseptic effects for a long time.

Licorice root is commonly used in herbal remedies because of its unique properties of harmonizing and softening any harshness and bitterness of herbs it is combined with, whether the herbs are warming, moist, or dry. It is an important antidote and temperer to a variety of toxic plants or extract alkaloids, including caffeine in coffee and nicotine in tobacco.

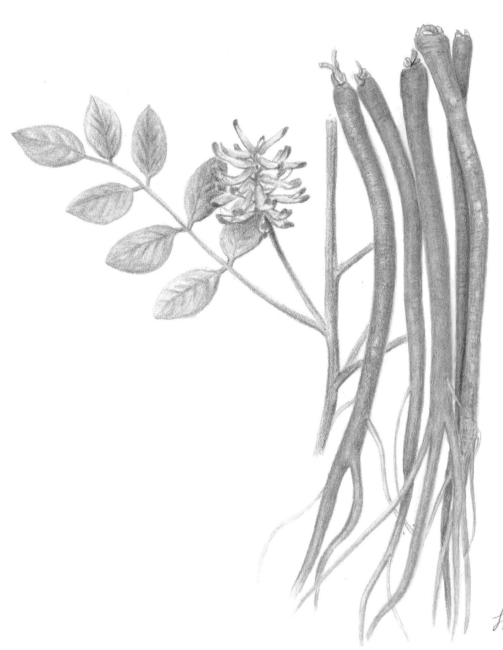

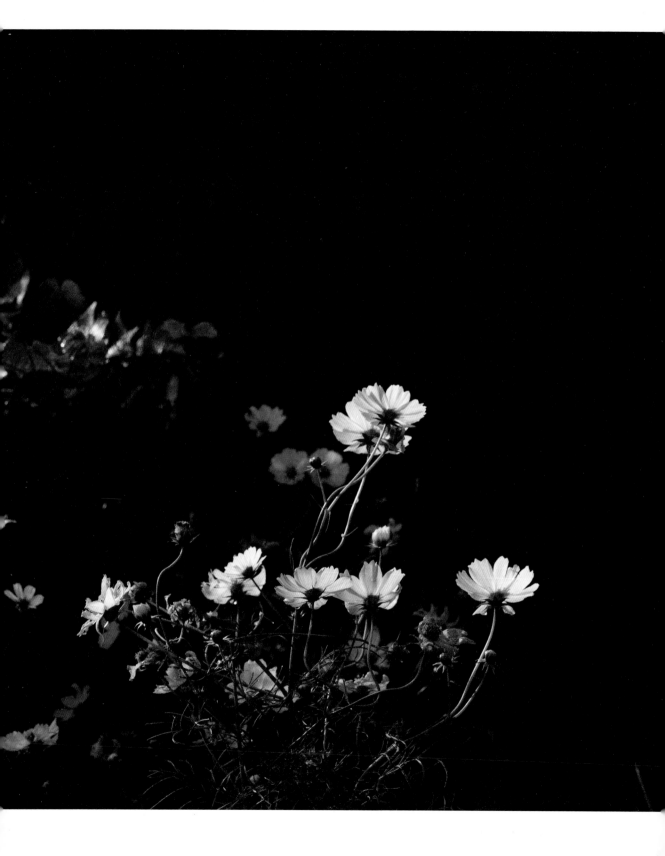

8 INFINITE BALANCE, PEACE, AND LONGEVITY

태극기 [taegeukgi]

Pearls of Wisdom
Conditions are pure and clean within this shell
Long periods of time and a rare find
A hidden pearl is a gift from nature (or mankind?)
Keep it.
Treasure it.
Never lose it.
Hold it close to your heart.

Confucius once said: If your plan is for one year, plant rice. If your plan is for ten years, plant trees. If your plan is for one hundred years, educate yourself and your children.

When we are curious to learn and understand from Mother Nature and others, we have everlasting knowledge that will be passed down for generations. Herbalists are stewards of the earth. When we meditate, grow, harvest, and produce, we are like a tree planted by streams of water, yielding fruit in season. Our leaves do not wither, yet they provide nutrients to the soil. Our work is all-consuming, and sharing our herbal knowledge and the fruits of our labor is required of us to live in our vital Qi.

We need pillars for strength and beauty in our practice so we can support the people around us who are burdened heavily. Here are the three pillars to keep in mind when building our Korean herbal apothecary:

- **Patience:** We are patient with our bodies as we need nutrients to sustain and improve our lives.
- **Joy and delight:** We are joyful when eating herbs that relish our senses and bring us delight.

- **Prevent or cure:** We prevent disease by mindfully consuming our everyday herbal meals and remedies, and we are cured from disease by the best medicine from Mother Nature as long as we stay consistent with our inner Qi.

PATIENCE

As I lie under a ginkgo tree, the fan-shaped leaves are waving at me.
The curly white clouds sail across the sky.
I am the daughter or son of Earth and Ocean.
Waves of blue in motion.
A warm fire within me.

Mung Meditation

멍 묵상 [mong mooksang]

Love takes patience, and as stewards of the earth, we must first be patient with ourselves before helping others. One of the ways to develop peaceful patience is through meditation. It is hard to disconnect from our modern world. We are constantly engaged with computers, phones, and all types of screens instead of connecting with nature. A daily practice of meditation, even for only five minutes, can make a drastic difference for our Qi and overall health, especially if your environment is frenetic, like living in a busy urban city.

Taking the time to meditate gives us more clarity and mindfulness. When we are more mindful of our actions, we make better decisions and improve our relationships with others. When our relationships with others are honed, then we create a safe space of trust, healing, and love. And when we have a safe space of trust, healing, and love, then transcendence comes upon us and we take care of our world.

Hitting mung is a form of meditation that's based on emptying our heart and mind to give our busy lives a break. Based on Buddhist principles of reaching a state

of "blankness," quieting the mind is a healthy practice in decreasing anxiety, stress, and depression. It restores our mind, body, and soul, and when we are in a blank state, there is an underlying sense of peace.

I breathe in the sky and thank Mother Nature for giving me this moment with ginkgo to clear my head and heart. I close my eyes and inhale a deep breath to cherish this moment. Then, I hit mung.

Wandering in the field of meditation, our chance should be to light upon the place of harvest. Herbs are energetic, and when we use them to make medicine, our energy and intention goes into the blends. Oh, let Mother Nature guide us to listen carefully to the people we make our medicine for and give honor and grace to the plants that are being used to heal.

Hands of Prayer and Healing

Once our mind is empty, we pray day and night for the people in our lives and for the world. Prayer may seem like a religious act, but the way I see it is having a conversation with our soul. We all have a soul, and when we pay attention to it, our soul usually guides us in the right direction. Our hands are energetic gifts when we place them together or raise them up to the sky. Let the energy of Mother Earth come inside through our hands.

We glean in the field after harvesting and amid the sheaves, we find love.

The love for our family, friends, lovers, animals, Mother Nature . . .

Qi is guiding our every step.

And each Qi step we take, we take a leap of faith and courage to experience a life unimaginable.

So seek and find an incredibly beautiful life of Qi.

Qi Steps: Making Changes with Patience and Kindness

Change is hard, so we have to make a choice to be ready and willing for change. Love and change takes patience, and if we love ourselves, we will be patient with the changes that we make.

Our dietary habits are not fixed. In my experience as a health coach, dietary changes are most difficult in the first ninety days. Just like a tortoise, it does not matter how slowly you progress, just as long as you do not stop. A simple way to measure your progress is to look at your plate and determine if you made good choices, consistent with your desire to change.

When your body starts feeling nourished, you will feel an urge to stay consistent with your eating habits. I recommend changes in three phases: add new seeds, supplant, and weed out. You can still eat some "cheat" foods on some weeks or on special occasions.

Phase 1: Add New Seeds

Start by paying attention to what you eat and trying new things. Being more mindful of your eating habits during the first nine weeks will gradually change your appetite, and you will start looking forward to the new more nutritious foods.

- Add fermented products, such as fermented soybean paste, miso, and kimchi, one or two days a week.
- Eat more fruits and vegetables, including pickled vegetables such as pickled soybeans or garlic. Have fresh vegetable juice or a smoothie.
- Include herbal teas, organic sesame seeds, and fresh, refrigerated flaxseed oil as part of your diet.
- Soak grains overnight before cooking them.
- Use extra-virgin olive oil for salad dressings and sesame or perilla oil for stir-frying.
- Enjoy sea vegetables, especially kelp, as a supplementary vegetable, condiment, or broth.
- Eat wild fish one or two days a week.

SIMPLE SMOOTHIE

One of my favorite smoothie blends is combining a bunch of spinach, half a banana, a teaspoon of matcha, a pitted jujube, a cup (235 ml) of almond milk, and a pinch of ginger powder.

Phase 2: Supplant

Now that you have added good seeds to your diet, begin shifting the emphasis of your diet toward more natural and less processed sources. These simple dietary changes emphasize vitamin- and mineral-rich whole foods.

- Increase the amount of organic fruits and vegetables in your diet. Choose fresh vegetables instead of canned or frozen vegetables.
- Add dairy-free or nut-based products instead of dairy products.
- Enjoy fresh-made vegetable juices or herbal teas instead of soft drinks and sweetened juices.
- Eat homemade soups instead of canned soups.
- Have porridges instead of bread and eat whole grains like barley, brown rice, and buckwheat.
- Continue to use olive oil or sesame oil instead of refined vegetable oils. Eat wild fish instead of other meats.
- Use honey or stevia instead of other sweeteners and substitute sea salt for table salt.

Phase 3: Weed Out

As you continue tending the new seeds of your diet, know that these changes can restore health. Some of the weeds may be persistent—and hard to let go of. Keep in mind that a healthy diet helps you prevent and overcome many functional diseases such fatigue, depression, and anxiety.

- Remove all forms of sugar and processed foods.

- Cut out refined sugars, vegetable oils, and deep-fried food.
- Avoid refined margarine and hydrogenated oils, caffeine, nicotine, and alcohol.

JOY AND DELIGHT

"Ahhh shewonhae!" Grandma said as she quenched the last drop of ginseng liquid gold, *samgyetang*, Korean ginseng chicken broth. We must experience third taste, *shewonhan mat* (시원한 맛), the pleasurable and delightful taste in our herbal remedies and foods.

Koreans experience *shewonhan mat* when drinking broths with proper herbal and fermented blends, which balances the salt concentration of the food and gives rise to a seasoning that hits *shewonhan mat*. The diverse sensations of food touching our mouth, swallowing the taste in our throat, and digesting it in our stomach gives us the joyful spectrum of colorful foods. This is the third taste.

Essence of Broths

The attributes of hot, warm, cool, or cold, and tastes of spicy, sweet, bitter, sour, or salty, blended in liquid gold create the yin and yang of Qi. With every Korean meal, there usually is a pot or bowl of herbal soup or stew.

Beef Broth

쇠고기 국물 [soegogi gukmul]

Sipping on a hot cup of bone broth is a great way to warm up during cold weather or if your body normally runs cold, as well as keeping our immune system healthy. Bone broth has been consumed for centuries, but is gaining more popularity because of its incredible health benefits.

Koreans consume bone broth year-round and are famous for ox bone soup called seolleongtang. Along with being rich in nutrients, this elixir is a great source of protein and amino acids that help your body produce collagen. Bone broth differs from regular chicken or beef stock as it usually is boiled for over sixteen hours compared with regular stock, which takes about four hours. The cooking process for bone broth is much longer; therefore, more nutrients from the animal bones and vegetables can be extracted into the stock. Incorporating nutrient-rich foods in your diet will help you boost your immune system for the upcoming fall and winter seasons. Bone broth provides essential vitamins and minerals, including vitamins A and K as well as calcium, magnesium, phosphorus, and iron.

The nutrients found in bone broth are also great for the gut—and a healthy gut is critical for an overall strong immune system. The long cooking time for bone broth allows collagen gelatin to be released from animal bones and ligaments. This makes bone broth a great elixir for those with digestive issues and leaky-gut syndrome. Collagen and gelatin can help restore and connect severed tissue in the gut and fight inflammation. Collagen is great for firming skin, strengthening joints, and reducing inflammation.

MAKING BONE BROTH

The key to making good broth is removing blood from the bones. Beef shank bones should be soaked in cold water to cleanse all the blood from the bones and then boiled. The bones are rinsed and boiled again in cold water. As the water is at a high boiling point, reduce it to medium and allow the bones to boil for at least 3 hours. Then, strain the broth using a cotton cloth. Allow it to cool until a layer of fat rises to the surface and then scrape it off.

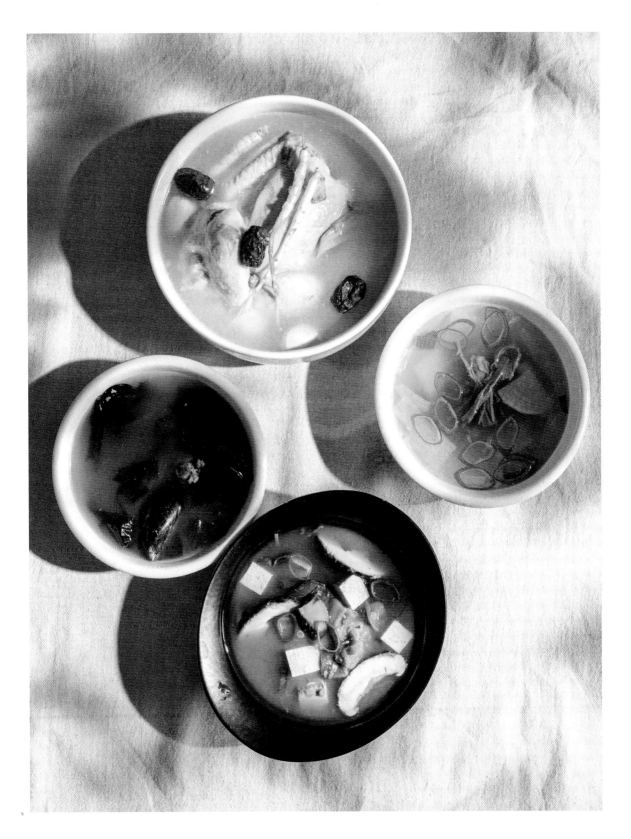

Bone broth may appear as just a new wellness trend, but our ancestors have been using bone as a staple of their diets for centuries. So, let's return to this ancient remedy for health support. Incorporating bone broth into your diet should not be too difficult as bone broth is delicious by itself. You could start your mornings with a hot cup of bone broth and Qi Alchemy herbal tea. This elixir is a great base for soups and noodles, and it is even being added to smoothies. Sipping on bone broth or adding it to recipes year-round will flavor your meals and benefit your body.

Chicken Broth

닭고기 국물 [dakgogi gukmul]

Rich in essential fatty acids and protein, chicken broth is a necessity. It is boiled in water for at least two hours with onion, garlic, scallions, black pepper, ginger, and rice wine. Chicken broth also contains selenium, which helps prevent and manage cardiovascular diseases, so someone with high cholesterol or has experienced a stroke should consume chicken broth. Make sure to strain the broth with a cotton cloth.

KOREAN GINSENG CHICKEN SOUP

인삼치료 비누 [insamchilyo binu]

SERVES 4

1 Cornish hen, approx-
   imately 1¼ pounds
   (570 g)
½ cup (90 g) sweet rice
1 ginseng root
5 dried jujubes
2 cloves garlic
1 onion, quartered
¼ teaspoon crushed
   ginger
5 cups (1.2 L) water
Salt and pepper, to taste
1 to 2 scallions, chopped

This herbaceous chicken soup, commonly known as the Korean penicillin, is a healing soup for those who are recovering from an illness or are under extreme levels of stress. It is used to restore Qi that's lost due to sickness. Indicated uses are for a weakened immune system, lack of appetite, stamina, chronic fatigue syndrome, depression, convalescence, and depression.

1. Thoroughly clean the Cornish hen. Wash the sweet rice and then drain it through a fine-mesh sieve. Stuff the rice, ginseng, jujubes, and garlic in the cavity of the Cornish hen.

2. Add the Cornish hen, onions, ginger, and water to a large stockpot. Cover and simmer over low heat for 2 to 3 hours until all the ingredients are cooked and tender.

3. Remove the Cornish hen from the broth and allow it to cool slightly. Gently pull off bite-size pieces of meat and add them to the broth. Season with salt and pepper and serve hot, garnished with scallions.

—

When we are depleted and need restoration, we drink our healing ginseng soup.

Seafood Broth

해산물 국물 [haesanmul gukmul]

This broth is an excellent source of minerals, and it often is used to make fermented soybean soup and many other seafood stews and soups. It is full of calcium and gelatin, so it is a great substitute for bone broth.

MAKING SEAFOOD BROTH

First, desalt the mussels or clams by soaking them in water and ½ cup (120 ml) of white vinegar for about 20 minutes. As the mussels breathe, they filter water and expel sand. Add the 1 pound (455 g) of mussels, 1 sheet of 3- by 3-inch (7.5 by 7.5 cm) kelp, 1 onion, 2 cloves of chopped garlic, ½ cup (120 ml) rice wine, and 12 cups (2.8 L) of water to a large stockpot. Boil over medium heat for at least 1 hour. Strain the broth with a cotton cloth.

Korean Vegetable Broth

한국 야채 국물 [hanguk yachae gukmul]

With vast health benefits, vegetable broth is full of antioxidants, strengthens bones, and improves skin health. It contains a large amount of vitamin A, which improves eye health.

MAKING KOREAN VEGETABLE BROTH

Korean vegetable broth usually includes radish, cabbage, shiitake mushroom, dashima (dried kelp), green onion roots, onion, and garlic. Shiitake and dashima are great sources of glutamic acid, an amino acid that enhances a savory taste and is full of nutrients. We initially bring the ingredients to a boil and then reduce the temperature to medium heat and simmer slowly to create a delicious and nutritious broth. Always strain the broth with a cotton cloth.

KOREAN RADISH SOUP

무국 [muguk]

SERVES 2

½ medium Korean radish
½ teaspoon chopped
  garlic
2 teaspoons sesame oil
1 piece dried dashima
  kelp/seaweed (about the
  size of an index card)
3 cups (700 ml) water
Salt and pepper, to taste
Cooked rice, for serving

Korean radish, mu (무), is an essential ingredient in soups, stews, broths, and even kimchi variations. It brings out a refreshing taste, and every part of the plant is used from the taproot to the greens. It is highly nutritious and contains folic acid, ascorbic acid, and potassium, and it is a good source of vitamin B_6, riboflavin, magnesium, copper, and calcium. It is a great way to clear out phlegm and eliminate bacteria and other pathogens. Mu contains the enzyme myrosinase, which helps break down starchy food in the digestive tract and also helps with detoxification. For a vegetarian or vegan soup, this radish soup recipe is a simple and nourishing meal with rice.

1. Cut the radish into circular tubes and then cut lengthwise and vertically to create rectangular-shaped slices.

2. In a stockpot, cook the garlic in sesame oil over low heat for 1 to 2 minutes. Add the radish and cook over low heat for 2 to 3 minutes. Add the seaweed and water to the stockpot and season with salt and pepper.

3. Cover and bring to a boil over medium-high heat. Reduce the heat and simmer for 15 minutes or until the radish is tender. Serve hot with a bowl of rice.

—

We need more mu in our lives. Not moo like a cow. Mu like radish.

Porridges

죽 [juk]

Compared with trendy green juices and kale salads, rice porridge may not immediately come to mind as a glamorous health food, but do not be fooled. Rice porridge is actually a quintessential and nutritious remedy in traditional Eastern medicine for troubled digestive systems and is very restorative.

Instead of eating toast in the morning, try juk (porridge) for a nutritious and savory rice porridge that's better than bread. There are many porridge varieties offered in Korea, from red beans to pumpkin. It is easy to digest and low carb, and it is very good for elderly people and those who are recuperating.

SAVORY RICE PORRIDGE

죽 [juk]

SERVES 4

RICE PORRIDGE
1 cup (168 g) mixed-grain rice
2 teaspoons sesame oil
2 cloves garlic, minced
1 piece (1 inch, or 2.5 cm) ginger
3 tablespoons (60 g) soybean paste
2 cups (475 ml) water
1½ cups (355 ml) vegetable broth

TOPPINGS
¼ cup (26 g) bean sprouts
1 soft-boiled egg
¼ cup (18 g) sliced mushrooms, sautéed
¼ cup (25 g) sliced kimchi
2 scallions, sliced
Black pepper, to taste
Sesame oil, to drizzle

Savory rice porridges in Asia are very common for breakfast or a light meal. Herbs and superfood ingredients such as ginger, sesame oil, and kimchi are often incorporated to enhance its medicinal properties and add flavor to the porridge.

1. Wash the rice and soak it in cold water for at least 30 minutes.

2. Heat a pot or saucepan over medium-high heat. Add the sesame oil, garlic, and ginger. Cook for 1 to 2 minutes, being careful not to burn the garlic.

3. Strain the rice through a fine-mesh sieve. Add it to the pot and stir for 3 to 4 minutes, until the rice is sticky. Add the soybean paste, water, and vegetable broth. Cook for 20 minutes over medium-high heat. Stir the porridge a few times and reduce the heat to low. Cover and cook for 10 minutes.

4. To serve: Pour the soup into bowls, add the toppings, and drizzle with sesame oil.

—

Juk is a universally nourishing food we consume to remind ourselves of the circle of life.

Pickled Herbs and Vegetables

Fermentation is a core practice in Korean culinary and herbalism. Pickling is fermentation with lactic-acid producing bacteria. It has benefits similar to those of fermenting milk to make yogurt. The bacteria predigest the plant constituents, freeing up minerals. The sour lactic acid also has health benefits of its own, helping to regulate the normal bacteria in the gut.

With its vibrant red color and bold spiciness, kimchi is the most famous pickled garnish associated with Korean cuisine. However, danmuji, known for being bright yellow, is a favorite fermented ingredient in Korean culture that also deserves the spotlight. Danmuji is pickled daikon radish and is a key ingredient in kimbap as well as a garnish to a variety of dishes, including Korean porridge. With a unique tangy flavor, pickled daikon radish adds complexity, texture, and a nutritional boost to any meal. Danmuji is easy to make and great to have in the fridge to elevate a plate, or simply eat it on its own.

Daikon radish is well-known for being a nutritional root vegetable. Low in calories, it also has an impressive amount of antioxidants, vitamins, and minerals. The root is rich in vitamin C, as well as a great source of calcium, magnesium, and potassium. Already loaded with nutritional benefits from the daikon radish, danmuji also contains gut-friendly probiotics from the fermentation process. The pickling period produces healthy microorganisms that help balance bacteria in the body. A healthy gut supports many of the body's functions, like maintaining a strong immune system.

Being pickled, danmuji has a unique sweet and sour taste. Seasoned with spices such as gochugaru (Korean red pepper flakes), sesame oil, sesame seeds, scallions, or even turmeric, danmuji can also be savory and spicy. Pickled daikon radishes are truly a versatile ingredient, accompanying kimbap, bibimbap, salads, and entrées. Danmuji is simple to make, only requiring daikon radishes, vinegar, a few spices, and patience during the pickling process. Danmuji can also be bought at Korean markets or Asian grocery stores in the refrigerated section, usually near the kimchi.

Fermented Foods

Kimchi originated over three thousand years ago and was created to preserve vegetables during the cold winter seasons in Korea. Unlike most fermented vegetables that are just seasoned with salt, kimchi has a unique fermentation process because it is mixed with a variety of herbs and spices such as garlic, red pepper, ginger, green onion, and fermented seafood seasoning. Although cabbage is the most commonly used base for kimchi, there are hundreds of kimchi varieties including lotus root, cucumber, wild chive, balloon flower root, burdock root, radish, perilla leaves, sweet potato vines, and more. Kimchi is frequently included in Korean cuisine.

There is a Korean saying, "Don't drink kimchi soup first." Koreans value their health, and one of the most important ways to look after our health is to manage our eating habits. Kimchi is used as a side dish for every meal, and kimchi soup is one of the most common spicy soups eaten after eating solid foods to improve digestion and help reduce bloating.

Kimchi is filled with nutrients such as vitamins A, B_1, B_2, and C. It promotes digestion, regulates cholesterol, aids weight management, boosts immune system, has antiaging and antioxidant properties, and helps prevent cancer. The lactic acid and lactobacillus found in kimchi also relieves hangovers.

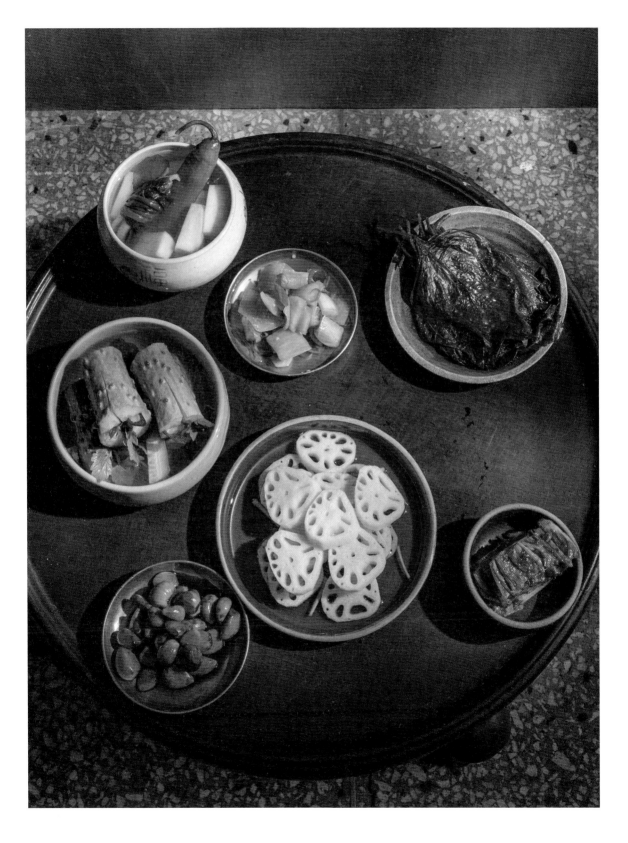

KIMCHI CAULIFLOWER FRIED RICE

SERVES 4

1 small head cauliflower
2 tablespoons (28 ml)
  olive oil
2 teaspoons perilla oil
2 teaspoons minced garlic
¼ cup (40 g) diced onion
⅓ cup (43 g) chopped
  carrots
⅓ cup (47 g) sliced
  shiitake mushroom
½ cup (50 g) kimchi
¼ cup (10 g) perilla
  leaves, chopped
3 tablespoons (45 ml) soy
  sauce
1 teaspoon gochujang
Cooked organic chicken
  or fried egg (optional)
2 scallions, thinly sliced

김치콜리플라워볶음밥 [gimchikollipeullawobokk-eumbab]

This is a modern twist on kimchi cauliflower rice.

1. Grate the cauliflower to make cauliflower rice. Add the olive oil, perilla oil, and garlic to a large frying pan over medium-low heat. Then, add the onions, carrots, cauliflower, and shiitake mushrooms. Once the vegetables are cooked, add the kimchi, perilla leaves, soy sauce, and gochujang.

2. Stir-fry everything over high heat until cooked through. Top the stir-fry with cooked organic chicken or a fried egg (if using) and garnish with scallions.

—

We are connected to everyone and everything. We are Qi.

TOMATO KIMCHI SAUCE

MAKES 1 PINT (473 ML)

1½ to 2 pounds (680
  to 900 kg) ripe grape
  tomatoes (or any variety
  you desire), halved
10 cloves garlic
2 tablespoons (28 ml)
  olive oil, plus more to
  drizzle
1 medium onion
2 cloves garlic, minced
10 ounces (280 g) kimchi
1½ teaspoons sea salt
1 teaspoon freshly
  ground black pepper

토마토 김치 소스 [tomato kimchi soseu]

Keep this simple yet versatile tomato sauce chunky for a great everyday dip or blend it until smooth to use when making pasta or pizza. Kimchi helps give it that extra kick.

1. Preheat the oven to 450°F (230°C, or gas mark 8). Arrange the tomatoes and garlic cloves in a single layer on a large baking sheet, making sure the tomatoes are facing cut-side up. Generously drizzle with olive oil and season with salt and pepper. Roast for 45 minutes until tender or they have browned.

2. Heat the oil in a large saucepan or Dutch oven over medium-high heat. Add the onion, minced garlic, and kimchi. Cook for 1 to 2 minutes, stirring, until fragrant. Add the roasted tomatoes and garlic, stir, and cook until the kimchi has softened. Remove from the heat and season with salt and pepper.

3. Transfer to a blender or use an immersion blender and blend until desired texture. Once cooled, transfer to an airtight container. The sauce can be kept chilled for up to 3 days or frozen for 1 month.

—

The passionate color of red enhances the sweetness of tomatoes and spiciness of Korean red chile peppers.

PREVENTION

The Path Unspoken
Treading carefully as we decide which path to take
Straight and narrow?
Circles and zig zags?
We want clarity and predictability by the path we choose
Everlasting peace unravels when we completely surrender
At the end, the path leads the same way.

Sleep

There is nothing like waking up feeling refreshed and rejuvenated after a terrific night of sleep. We might take it for granted, but sleep is an important time when we restore the mind and body, making it vital for our Qi. When we have trouble falling asleep or staying asleep, it can be extremely frustrating. Not only do we wake up feeling fatigue, but continuous lack of sleep can cause weight gain and mood changes, affect hormones, and lower your immunity. Clearly, we need to prioritize sleep.

In South Korea, nap competitions are organized to promote awareness of sleep deprivation and its effects on health. To encourage Koreans to focus on their rest, the competition awards the individual who has the longest and deepest sleep.

We are living in stressful and uncertain times, and when the mind is racing with so many worries, it is nearly impossible to have quality sleep. With a few tips and techniques, you will be able to receive the restorative rest you need and deserve.

To feel a sense of calm, turning screens off is extremely helpful. It is easy to switch channels, but it is difficult when we also have access to it on our mobile devices. For a limit on news and social media, it is prudent to turn off your phone in the evening. The news, texts, and social media will only add to your worries and can even cause anxiety. We are responsible for our lives, so cutting out our devices to relax and focus on ourselves is a prudent daily practice. Two

hours before bed or even thirty minutes, pick up a book, take a bath, or meditate to help unwind.

If you are still worrying about the days ahead while you are trying to fall asleep, make a to-do list for the next day and also write down what's concerning. Writing the items and your feelings out on paper makes them appear more manageable. It is better to have them on paper than spinning in your head all night.

While we limit screen time, setting a nighttime ritual will help your body know it is time to relax and prepare for bed. After turning off the news and setting aside your devices, find what brings you peace. That could be reading a good book, taking a bath, doing yoga, or meditating. Herbal tea is a great addition to any evening routine. Qi Alchemy's herbal pearls are versatile and can be taken either in the morning or in the evening. The proprietary blend of herbs helps ease tension and relaxes muscles, making it a perfect remedy to de-stress. Maintaining this routine also helps put your body on a schedule of knowing it is almost time to sleep.

Creating a peaceful sleep environment can make a huge difference. Limit clutter around your bed so your mind doesn't feel disordered as well. Aromatherapy and essential oils can also add to a sense of peace in your bedroom. One of my favorite herbal oils is frankincense because of its long healing history and its sweet woody and citrus notes. Placing a few drops into your hands and inhaling it before sleeping is an amazing way to relieve stress. In addition, making your room a temperature that suits your body temperature can be beneficial in the process of falling asleep.

Daily activity is crucial for your health and for the quality of your sleep. Exercise tires you out and also reduces stress, making it easier to fall asleep, so try to exercise during the day.

It seems obvious but it is important to steer clear of caffeine at least six hours before bed. Drinking too much caffeine will have us tossing and turning all night. Instead, turn to decaffeinated tea that will help soothe the mind and body.

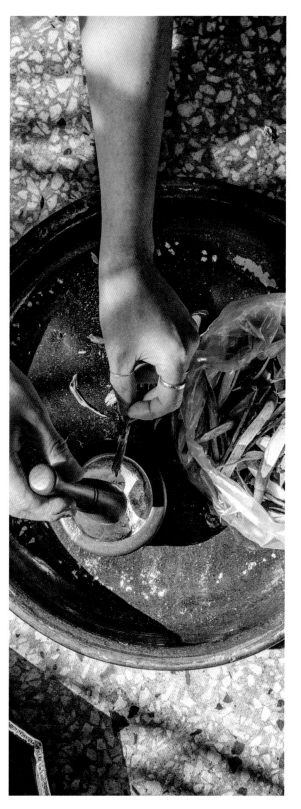

Ceremony

May things be just like hangawi, no more, no less.

Hangawi (한가위), a full harvest moon, is a time of abundance and giving thanks to our ancestors. Herbalism is ceremonial, and as we follow the lunar calendar, we honor our ancestors by offering harvested crops and fruit. We give gratitude to our ancestors and to Mother Nature.

We also give gifts of herbal pearls to our loved ones. The pearl-like herbal blends, known as hwan in Korea, were created during the Joseon dynasty by royal physicians in the 1300s. Whenever we feel any pain or discomfort, we take herbal pearls, and on special occasions, we take moon pearls that are coated in gold. The gift of herbs is a gift of health and longevity.

One of my favorite ceremonies is giving a Korean tea ceremony because meditation tea is a form of meditation in and of itself. A Buddhist monk, Dalma, brought tea to Korea. Dalma tried very hard to practice meditation, but he would constantly fall asleep. Frustrated with himself, he cut off his eyelids and threw them on the ground. The eyelids transformed and blossomed into a tea plant. Dalma then made tea from the leaves, drank it, and was able to stay awake while meditating.

Every country is influenced by its natural environment. China is surrounded by huge mountains and vast fields. Japan has flat lands and a big mountain in the middle. Korea has smaller mountains and narrow fields. Gardens play an important role in how citizens see their relationship with nature, and tea culture resembles the garden of each country. China's tea ceremony uses gestures that are lavish and elaborate. Japan's tea ceremony uses movement in a minimalistic and efficient way. Korea's tea ceremony resembles nature—free and smooth—as we have come midway between Chinese and Japanese cultures and metamorphosed into our own unique culture.

Teas gives rise to four kinds of thought for Korean Buddhists. They are respectfulness, peacefulness, purity, and quietness. Those teas that bring out more of these thoughtful qualities are revered. Most teas should be consumed as fresh as possible.

> *Father lined us up like a line of daisies*
> *We have a serious problem.*
> *We have a drought...*
> *The letter B was written on one of our report cards.*
> *In America B means Baseline.*
> *In Korea B means Bad.*
>
> *What is the solution to our drought problem?*
> *To pay attention to the wilted daisy...*
>
> *So father got his bamboo stick and hit the other daisies on the wrist*
> *Because they were responsible for the wilting daisy.*

Love can be painful at times, and some of the purest forms of love is revealing the truth to someone who does not see their truth. Building a community of friends that are like family takes much time and effort, but it is worth growing a garden together, harvesting together, and tasting the fruits of our labor together.

Kimchi Community

One of the ways we labor together with our community is a tradition called kimjang, the making and sharing of kimchi. In the spring, each household ferments seafood called saewoo jeot (새우젓), fermented shrimp and anchovies with salt. In the summer, we buy thousand-day sea salt, which brings the mineral-packed taste with larger crystals and is used to preserve fermented foods for two to three years until its bitter taste is gone. In the late summer, red peppers are dried and ground into powder to season kimchi. In the late fall, the women of the home consider the weather conditions and decide the date for making kimchi. Traditional and new techniques and ideas are shared and accumulated through the custom of sharing kimchi. This custom helps foster community, as family members in the local village gather together to harvest and make kimchi.

The unity and creator of all things is Love and everything in all its infinite splendor, whether it be a flower or the earth, a dewdrop or star, they are all manifestations of Love. As we come together, we bow to our ancestors and Mother Earth for protection, wisdom, and guidance as we live purposefully and spread our seeds with Love.

REFERENCES

Bode AM, Dong Z. "The Amazing and Mighty Ginger." In *Herbal Medicine: Biomolecular and Clinical Aspects*, 2nd ed., eds. Benzie IFF, Wachtel-Galor S. Boca Raton, FL: CRC Press/Taylor & Francis, 2011. https://www.ncbi.nlm.nih.gov/books/NBK92775/.

Centers for Disease Control and Prevention. "The Role of Sodium in Your Food." https://www.cdc.gov/salt/role_of_sodium.htm.

Chang HL, Young K, Yang SK, Young Y. "Ancestral Ritual Food of Korean *Jongka*: Historical Changes of the Table Setting." *Journal of Ethnic Foods*. 2018; 5(2):121–132. https://www.sciencedirect.com/science/article/pii/S235261811830091X.

Classified Collection of Medical Formulas (Euibang Yuchui), published by the Joseon government in 1477.

Dhyani A, Chopra R, Garg M. "A Review on Nutritional Value, Functional Properties and Pharmacological Application of Perilla (Perilla Frutescens L.)." *Biomedical and Pharmacology Journal*. 2019;12(2).

Elpel TJ. *Botany in a Day: The Patterns Method of Plant Identification: Thomas J. Elpel's Herbal Field Guide to Plant Families*, rev. ed. Pony, MT: HOPS Press, 2004.

Institute of Medicine (US) Committee on Strategies to Reduce Sodium Intake. "Taste and Flavor Roles of Sodium in Foods: A Unique Challenge to Reducing Sodium Intake." In *Strategies to Reduce Sodium Intake in the United States*, eds. Henney JE, Taylor CL, Boon CS. Washington, DC: National Academies Press, 2010. https://www.ncbi.nlm.nih.gov/books/NBK50958/.

Kang SA, Oh HJ, Jang DJ, Kim MJ, Kwon DY. "*Siwonhan-mat*: The Third Taste of Korean Foods." *Journal of Ethnic Foods*. 2016 Mar;3(1):61–68. doi: https://doi.org/10.1016/j.jef.2016.02.004. https://www.sciencedirect.com/science/article/pii/S2352618116300075.

Kawatra P, Rajagopalan R. "Cinnamon: Mystic Powers of a Minute Ingredient." *Pharmacognosy Research*. 2015 Jun;7(Suppl 1):S1-6. doi: 10.4103/0974-8490.157990. PMID: 26109781; PMCID: PMC4466762. https://www.ncbi.nlm.nih.gov/pmc/articles/PMC4466762/.

Li H, Zhang X, Gu L, Li Q, Ju Y, Zhou X, Hu M, Li Q. "Anti-Gout Effects of the Medicinal Fungus *Phellinus igniarius* in Hyperuricaemia and Acute Gouty Arthritis Rat Models." *Frontiers in Pharmacology*. 2022 Jan 11;12:801910. doi: 10.3389/fphar.2021.801910. PMID: 35087407; PMCID: PMC8787200. https://www.ncbi.nlm.nih.gov/pmc/articles/PMC8787200/.

Memorial Sloan Kettering Cancer Center. "Chaga Mushroom: Purported Benefits, Side Effects & More." https://www.mskcc.org/cancer-care/integrative-medicine/herbs/chaga-mushroom.

Newman T. "What Are the Benefits of Garlic?" MedicalNewsToday. https://www.medicalnewstoday.com/articles/265853.

Nhất H. *The Heart of the Buddha's Teaching: Transforming Suffering into Peace, Joy & Liberation: The Four Noble Truths, the Noble Eightfold Path, and Other Basic Buddhist Teachings*. New York: Broadway Books, 1999.

Pullar JM, Carr AC, Vissers MCM. "The Roles of Vitamin C in Skin Health." *Nutrients*. 2017 Aug 12;9(8):866. doi: 10.3390/nu9080866. PMID: 28805671; PMCID: PMC5579659. https://www.ncbi.nlm.nih.gov/pmc/articles/PMC5579659/.

Rempel V, Fuchs A, Hinz S, Karcz T, Lehr M, Koetter U, Müller CE. "Magnolia Extract, Magnolol, and Metabolites: Activation of Cannabinoid CB2 Receptors and Blockade of the Related GPR55." *ACS Medicinal Chemistry Letters*. 2012 Nov 14;4(1):41-5. doi: 10.1021/ml300235q. PMID: 24900561; PMCID: PMC4027495. https://www.ncbi.nlm.nih.gov/pmc/articles/PMC4027495/#:~:text=The%20bark%20of%20Magnolia%20officinalis,sleeping%20disorders%2C%20and%20allergic%20diseases.

Sasangmedicine. "The Yin Type B (So Eum) Body Type." http://sasangmedicine.com/about-so-eum.html.

Schagen SK, Zampeli VA, Makrantonaki E, Zouboulis CC. "Discovering the Link Between Nutrition and Skin Aging." *Dermato-Endocrinology.* 2012 Jul 1;4(3):298-307. doi: 10.4161/derm.22876. PMID: 23467449; PMCID: PMC3583891. https://www.ncbi.nlm.nih.gov/pmc/articles/PMC3583891/.

Skenderi, Gazmend. *Herbal Vade Mecum: 800 Herbs, Spices, Essential Oils, Lipids, Etc., Constituents, Properties, Uses, and Caution.* Rutherford, NJ: Herbacy Press, 2003.

Tabassum NE et al. "*Ginkgo Biloba*: A Treasure of Functional Phytochemicals with Multimedicinal Applications." *Evidence-Based Complementary and Alternative Medicine.* 2022 Feb 28;2022:8288818. doi: 10.1155/2022/8288818. PMID: 35265150; PMCID: PMC8901348. https://www.ncbi.nlm.nih.gov/pmc/articles/PMC8901348/.

Timeless Classic Books. *The Sayings of Confucius.* CreateSpace Independent Publishing Platform, October 29, 2010.

Ware, M. "What Are the Health Benefits of Chives?" MedicalNewsToday. https://www.medicalnewstoday.com/articles/275009.

WebMD. "Chicken Broth: Are There Health Benefits?" https://www.webmd.com/diet/health-benefits-chicken-broth.

Yoo J, Lee E, Kim C, Lee J, Lixing L. "Sasang Constitutional Medicine and Traditional Chinese Medicine: A Comparative Overview." *Evidence-Based Complementary and Alternative Medicine.* 2012;2012:980807. doi: 10.1155/2012/980807. Epub 2011 Sep 19. PMID: 21941592; PMCID: PMC3176432. https://www.ncbi.nlm.nih.gov/pmc/articles/PMC3176432/.

Yoon, Grace. "7 Tips for Better Sleep." Qi Alchemy. June 23, 2020. https://www.qialchemy.com/blogs/koreanwellness/7-tips-for-falling-asleep.

Yoon, Grace. "A Definitive Guide to Korean Porridge." Qi Alchemy. August 18, 2021. https://www.qialchemy.com/blogs/koreanwellness/a-definitive-guide-to-korean-porridge#:~:text=Compared%20to%20trendy%20green%20juices,Medicine%20for%20troubled%20digestive%20systems.

Yoon, Grace. "Benefits of Bone Broth." Qi Alchemy. November 1, 2019. https://www.qialchemy.com/blogs/koreanwellness/benefits-of-bone-broth.

Yoon, Grace. "Benefits of Gingko Biloba." Qi Alchemy. August 27, 2022. https://www.qialchemy.com/blogs/koreanwellness/benefits-of-gingko-biloba.

Yoon, Grace. "Why You Should Be Eating Korean Pickled Radish." Qi Alchemy. October 1, 2021. https://www.qialchemy.com/blogs/koreanwellness/why-you-should-be-eating-korean-pickled-radish.

Zhao H, Feng Y-L, Wang M, Wang J-J, Liu T, Yu J. "The *Angelica dahurica*: A Review of Traditional Uses, Phytochemistry and Pharmacology." *Frontiers in Pharmacology.* 2022 July. doi: 10.3389/fphar.2022.896637. https://www.frontiersin.org/articles/10.3389/fphar.2022.896637/full#B37.

Zi L, Wu J, C, H, *Tao The Ching.* Boulder, CO: Shambhala, 1990.

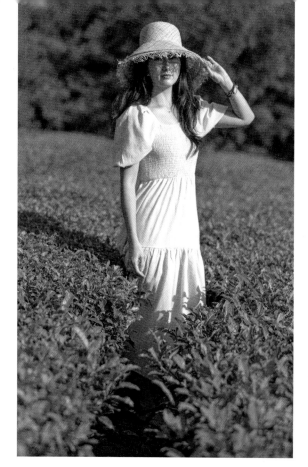

ACKNOWLEDGMENTS

I am grateful to Jill Alexander for choosing me to write this book about Korean herbalism.

Deep gratitude to the creatives, Michelle Min and Jane Kwan, who put so much heart and Seoul into the artwork. I also thank Samuel Marks for guiding and encouraging me to expand my wings. Thank you to Stephanie and Paul Kwon for believing in my mission to share Korean culture in a different light.

I have been encouraged by many herbalists and Eastern medicine doctors like Dr. Jun and Dr. Paek—thank you for giving me an opportunity to learn from you and share Korean herbal wisdom with the world.

My family (Yoo Jong Yoon, Eun Ju Yoon, Sara Yoon, Joanne Yoon) and Korean ancestors have given me so much love and grace throughout the years, and I am forever grateful for your support.

Finally, to our plants, thank you for giving us unconditional life and nourishment. We are stewards of Mother Earth.

ABOUT THE AUTHOR

GRACE YOON is an herbalist, certified health coach, and founder of Qi Alchemy, a Korean herbal wellness line bridging ancient Korean medicinal wisdom to the modern world. As a Korean American, she combines her knowledge of Korean herbalism, traditional medicine, nutrition science, and plant-based remedies for those seeking connection between ancient medicinal knowledge and modern life. She and Qi Alchemy have been featured in *Vogue*, *Forbes*, mindbodygreen, *Women's Wear Daily*, Coveteur, and Bloomberg.

Grace is deeply passionate about food and nutrition policy, regenerative farming, functional health, meditation, and environmental causes.

INDEX

THE KOREAN

HERBAL

APOTHECARY

Ancient Wisdom for
Wellness and Balance
in the Modern World

Grace Yoon

Quarto.com

© 2023 Quarto Publishing Group USA Inc.
Text © 2023 Grace Yoon
Photos © 2023 Michelle K. Min
Illustrations © 2023 Jane Kwan

First Published in 2023 by Fair Winds Press, an imprint of The Quarto Group,
100 Cummings Center, Suite 265-D, Beverly, MA 01915, USA.
T (978) 282-9590 F (978) 283-2742

Fair Winds Press titles are also available at discount for retail, wholesale, promotional, and bulk purchase. For details, contact the Special Sales Manager by email at specialsales@quarto.com or by mail at The Quarto Group, Attn: Special Sales Manager, 100 Cummings Center, Suite 265-D, Beverly, MA 01915, USA.

28 27 26 25 24   1 2 3 4 5

ISBN: 978-0-7603-8269-1

Digital edition published in 2023
eISBN: 978-0-7603-8270-7

Library of Congress Cataloging-in-Publication Data is available.

Cover design: Tanya Jacobson, tanyajacobson.co
Photography: Michelle K. Min, except pages 6, 60, 204 Qi Alchemy
Photography styling: Inock Jeon
Illustration: Jane Kwan, except pages 14, 15, 17, and 21 Esté Hupp

Printed in China

The information in this book is for educational purposes only. It is not intended to replace the advice of a physician or medical practitioner. Please see your healthcare provider before beginning any new health program. Check with your healthcare provider before starting any herbal regiment, especially if pregnant, to prevent any counterindications.